A Beginner's Guide to Intensive Care Medicine

A Beginner's Guide to Intensive Care Medicine

Edited by

SHONDIPON LAHA

BM BCh MA FRCA
Consultant in Anaesthesia and Intensive Care Medicine
Lancashire Teaching Hospitals NHS Foundation Trust

and

NITIN ARORA

MBBS MRCP(UK) FRCA
Specialty Registrar in Anaesthesia and Intensive Care Medicine
Lancashire Teaching Hospitals NHS Foundation Trust

Foreword by

JONATHAN GOODALL

Regional Adviser in ICM
NW Deanery

Radcliffe Publishing
Oxford • New York

Radcliffe Publishing Ltd
18 Marcham Road
Abingdon
Oxon OX14 1AA
United Kingdom

www.radcliffepublishing.com
Electronic catalogue and worldwide online ordering facility.

British Library Cataloguing in Publication Data
A catalogue record for this book is available from the British Library.

ISBN-13: 978 184619 451 1   .

Typeset by Pindar NZ, Auckland, New Zealand
Printed and bound by Cadmus Communications, USA

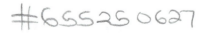

Contents

Foreword

Intensive care medicine (ICM) is an exciting, dynamic and rapidly evolving new specialty. It is both clinically rewarding and intellectually stimulating, but it can also be very bewildering for the uninitiated.

Those of us who have worked in the specialty have a tendency to forget how alien the environment of the intensive care unit can seem – how the machines and monitors that we embrace to guide clinical decision making appear an insurmountable hurdle to the novice intensivist. Trainees need reassurance that they have the clinical skills to work in this new clinical setting – that the patients are the same, they are assessed in the same way and that treatment will follow familiar principles.

Dr Laha and his colleagues have produced an excellent text, which will allay many of the fears and challenges that face those new to ICM. The authors start with a 'typical' day in ICM, and the essentials of assessing the critically ill patient. This 'back to basics' approach not only provides a clinical framework for new trainees, but also reminds them of similarities between ICM and other disciplines. This element of familiarity will reassure trainees, and it provides an excellent foundation for their ongoing education in the specialty. The book is divided into short, easy-to-read chapters, which are well planned and cover all the essentials of ICM. Chapters on 'What to do if the endotracheal tube or tracheostomy falls out' and 'Initial management of the patient with burns' include practical advice for trainees who may have limited knowledge and skills in these areas. The inclusion of chapters on communication and organ donation effectively demonstrates that ICM is more than invasive monitoring and organ replacement.

This book is an accessible, concise and practical guide to the first weeks in ICM. As time available for training in the workplace is reduced, doctors need all the help they can get when starting a new specialty. Shondipon Laha and his colleagues have produced a text that trainees will not only learn from, but will also enjoy reading. I am sure that more than a few trainers will find it useful, too!

Jonathan Goodall
Regional Adviser in ICM
NW Deanery
October 2010

Preface

The introduction of Modernising Medical Careers and the Foundation Programme for junior doctors has resulted in a refreshing change in the type of doctors who rotate to work on an intensive care unit. Prior to this, we were used to all trainees having completed at least their first year as a pre-registration house officer, and frequently senior house officer posts in medicine, surgery, anaesthesia or emergency medicine.

We now see foundation year 1 and 2 and acute care common stem trainees rotate to the unit. Added to this mix are the demands of the European Working Time Directive, resulting in the training of enthusiastic but inexperienced doctors.

Many of these doctors have found the current crop of medical textbooks on intensive care medicine intimidating, and have resorted to textbooks designed for other healthcare professionals.

The present book was designed to fill this gap. It is not a replacement for the traditional textbooks, but rather it adopts a pragmatic approach to common problems on the unit for both doctors and other allied healthcare workers.

Shondipon Laha
Nitin Arora
October 2010

About the editors

Dr Shondipon Laha BM BCh MA FRCA is a consultant in anaesthesia and intensive care medicine at Lancashire Teaching Hospitals NHS Foundation Trust. He read medicine at Oxford University and completed dual specialty training in anaesthesia and intensive care medicine in the North West of England.

Dr Nitin Arora MBBS MRCP(UK) FRCA has worked in medicine, intensive care and anaesthesia in India and the UK. He is a specialty registrar in anaesthesia and intensive care in the North West of England.

List of contributors

Dr Steven Benington
Specialist Registrar in Anaesthesia and Intensive Care Medicine
North West Rotation

Dr Peter Bunting
Consultant in Anaesthesia and Intensive Care Medicine
Lancashire Teaching Hospitals NHS Foundation Trust

Dr Harry Chan
Specialist Registrar in Anaesthesia and Intensive Care Medicine
North West Rotation

Dr Irfan Chaudry
Consultant in Anaesthesia and Intensive Care Medicine
Lancashire Teaching Hospitals NHS Foundation Trust

Mike Dickinson
Human Patient Simulator Training Coordinator
Lancashire Teaching Hospitals NHS Foundation Trust

Dr Ian Donaldson
Consultant in Anaesthesia and Intensive Care Medicine
Lancashire Teaching Hospitals NHS Foundation Trust

Dr Peter Duncan
Consultant in Anaesthesia and Intensive Care Medicine
Lancashire Teaching Hospitals NHS Foundation Trust

Dr Andrew Haughton
Consultant in Anaesthesia and Intensive Care Medicine
Lancashire Teaching Hospitals NHS Foundation Trust

Dr Anita Jeh
Foundation Trainee
Lancashire Teaching Hospitals NHS Foundation Trust

Dr Brendan McGrath
Consultant in Anaesthesia and Intensive Care Medicine
University Hospital of South Manchester NHS Foundation Trust

Dr Kenneth McGrattan
Consultant in Anaesthesia and Intensive Care Medicine
Lancashire Teaching Hospitals NHS Foundation Trust

Dr Shelley Newman
Specialty Trainee in Acute Care Common Stem Medicine
North West Rotation

Dr Thomas Owen
Consultant in Anaesthesia and Intensive Care Medicine
Lancashire Teaching Hospitals NHS Foundation Trust

Dr Mark Pugh
Consultant in Anaesthesia and Intensive Care Medicine
Lancashire Teaching Hospitals NHS Foundation Trust

Dr Rachel Saxon
Foundation Trainee
Lancashire Teaching Hospitals NHS Foundation Trust

Dr Amanda Shaw
Consultant in Anaesthesia and Intensive Care Medicine
Lancashire Teaching Hospitals NHS Foundation Trust

Dr Benjamin Slater
Specialist Registrar in Anaesthesia and Intensive Care Medicine
North West Rotation

Dr Dawn Soo
Specialty Trainee in Acute Care Common Stem Medicine
North West Rotation

Dr Craig Spencer
Consultant in Anaesthesia and Intensive Care Medicine
Lancashire Teaching Hospitals NHS Foundation Trust

Dr Michael Stewart
Specialty Trainee in Acute Care Common Stem Medicine
North West Rotation

Dr Jonathan Taylor
Foundation Trainee
Lancashire Teaching Hospitals NHS Foundation Trust

Dr Serena Tolhurst-Cleaver
Acute Medicine Specialty Trainee
North West Rotation

Dr Huw Twamley
Consultant in Anaesthesia and Intensive Care Medicine
Lancashire Teaching Hospitals NHS Foundation Trust

Dr James Wilson
Specialty Trainee in Anaesthesia and Intensive Care Medicine
North West Rotation

Acknowledgements

We would both like to thank all of the nursing and medical staff on the Critical Care Unit at Lancashire Teaching Hospitals NHS Foundation Trust.

Thanks to Mum, Dad and Shilpi for all the support over the years. And to my wife Alex, without whose encouragement it would have been impossible to create this book. And to Jonny and Ned – the laughter puts it all into perspective!

Shondipon Laha

Thanks to my wife Ira for her support and encouragement.

Nitin Arora

Your first day

Jonathan Taylor and Shondipon Laha

For the uninitiated, walking into the intensive care unit (ICU) can be an overwhelming experience. At first glance, with all the tubes, wires, machines and random beeps, it can seem a completely alien environment to that with which one is comfortable, on the main hospital wards. However, closer inspection reveals that the majority of what happens in the ICU is not very different to what goes on anywhere else in the hospital – it just looks that way!

By its very nature, an ICU will contain some of a hospital's sickest patients, and this thought alone is enough to scare away even some of the most battle-hardened consultants from its doors. Again, on closer inspection, this proves to be true only to some extent. Unlike almost any other hospital ward, the ICU has a vetted cohort of patients, whereas medical wards will have little or no say in which patients are admitted through their doors. With few exceptions, before a patient is admitted to the ICU their history and, where possible, the patient will have been examined to assess the appropriateness of admission. These assessments will factor in a number of variables, in an attempt to answer a few basic questions. These include the following:

- What is the diagnosis?
- What can the ICU achieve that cannot be achieved on the ward?

- Is the condition reversible?'
- Is ICU admission in the best interest of the patient?

As with any decision as to how aggressively patient management should be pursued, a number of ethical dilemmas are faced when denying admission (and conversely when admitting patients when aggressive therapy is probably not in their best interest), and conflicting opinions among staff are a frequent occurrence when making patient management decisions, which can present a significant (if not the most significant) challenge to the new doctor.

A common misconception about intensive care is that what goes on within the specialty, and the interventions that are performed, are almost a form of witchcraft, and beyond the capability of most other wards or specialties. However, as with the unit itself, closer inspection reveals that this is also a misconception. The overriding principle of intensive care is not to perform complex interventions or investigations, but to aggressively support the patient's organ systems. The backbone of the care that patients receive on an ITU is, as with all acute medicine, ABCDE (airway, breathing, circulation, disability, exposure), as has been drummed into each medical professional ever since student days.

Often one of the most daunting aspects of an ICU to the novice is the amount of unfamiliar equipment that surrounds each patient's bed space (which itself will often be several times larger than a typical ward bed space, mostly to accommodate the equipment!), ranging from ventilators, and myriad wires, lines and tubes, to various items of invasive and non-invasive monitoring equipment. Each of these will also, apparently constantly, be emitting some form of alarm – the intensity and serious-sounding nature of which often in no way correlates with the severity of what it is indicating. For example, a syringe driver that has reached the end of infusion may emit a loud two-tone alarm, whereas a disconnected ventilator may only produce an asthmatic wheeze! As a novice, you will often find yourself jumping at every minor sound, thinking that each of these requires you to spring into action. However, this is rarely the case, and until you learn to differentiate between each of the sounds, a useful approach is to pay attention to how nursing and experienced medical staff are reacting to the various alarms, and to follow their lead.

Similarly, as medical professionals, from the first day of our training it is drummed into us to 'listen to the patient, he is telling you the diagnosis.'

However, a significant proportion of ICU patients will be intubated and/ or sedated, so recognising evolving situations will require much more reliance on clinical acumen and ability to interpret what the many measured parameters are telling you. Again, for those who are not experienced in working in an ICU setting, this can be a somewhat overwhelming task, and later chapters of this book will aim to assist you in developing a systematic, methodical approach that will enable you to decipher what the numbers are telling you. As with any other setting, although perhaps even more so on the ICU, you are surrounded by many experienced staff who will in most cases be able to give you invaluable assistance. This makes intensive care medicine a multi-disciplinary specialty in the truest sense of the phrase, with diagnoses and management options often being the result of the collated expertise of many individuals from varied specialties.

The 'typical' day

Most days will start with the morning handover, and for those of you from general medical or surgical backgrounds this may come as a shock – 'handover' is not just a term to describe the day staff arriving and night staff going home! The ICU handover will ideally involve all of the day and night medical staff, along with key nursing and allied staff, and will aim to give a complete overview of each patient, detailing matters of concern and significant changes through each shift. It is not uncommon for this process to last well over 30 minutes, depending on the unit size and dependency (essentially a measure of the number of patients and the required nursing intensity). It represents a crucial part of the day, as the ICU provides continuous 24/7 care, and most patients will have issues that require continuous review, or there may be jobs that need to be carried on across shift changes.

Following handover, patients on the unit will be divided among the junior staff who then undertake detailed daily reviews, which are covered in the following chapter, and complete urgent jobs as necessary. In addition, one or more of the junior staff will take referral calls from wards and external sources. This often requires that they forego their immediate responsibilities for unit patient reviews to assess ward patients, a process which may not uncommonly take up most of the time allocated for daily reviews. It is therefore important that staff remain flexible and work closely to ensure that all unit patients receive adequate review.

Being responsible for reviewing ward referrals can also often be an intimidating prospect for the uninitiated, and it is advisable to take opportunities early on to review patients with another more experienced doctor to get a feel for which criteria are used in determining suitability for ITU admission.

Following the completion of daily reviews and urgent jobs, a consultant-led ward round will usually take place, where each patient is presented, and decisions regarding alteration of the management plan are typically made depending on the evolving picture and new information elicited during the daily review. On completion of the ward round, any outstanding and new jobs from the ward round should be completed before the end of the shift and handover to the late shift.

Although the above outline of a typical day may suggest that not very much happens during the average day shift, it should not take long to realise the level of detail required in reviewing and rounding patients, and the time that is needed to complete complex, intricate procedures and the many other daily tasks, including discussion with families, liaising with other hospital departments and teams, and chasing results, among numerous other jobs. You will find that the hours quickly slip away!

Finally, the most important thing to remember when undertaking a placement on the ITU is to enjoy yourself. The opportunities to gain experience in perfecting practical, communication and decision-making skills are almost second to none. The same is true of supervision and teaching opportunities, which will often be considerably greater than in any ward-based specialties. If you take full advantage of these opportunities you will have an intense but ultimately extremely rewarding experience.

2

The daily review of a patient

Shondipon Laha

This is an important aspect of intensive care. Many of these patients have complex comorbidities and pathology, and a systematic method of assessing them allows problems to be broken down and a management plan to be instituted.

Primary diagnosis
- The reason for admission (e.g. pneumonia).

Background and progress
- A summary of the patient's past medical history and the history of this admission, followed by what has happened over the course of their ICU stay.

Problems during the last 24 hours
- A summary of any problems or improvements that have occurred since the last review.

Respiratory system
- Examination of the respiratory system.

- Is the patient intubated or do they have a tracheostomy? If so, what type and size of tube has been used?
- How are they being ventilated and what are the settings?
- Amount and characteristics of any sputum.
- Oxygen saturation and arterial blood gas analysis.
- When was the last chest X-ray performed and what did it show?
- Is the patient on any respiratory medication?

Cardiovascular system

- Palpation of pulses.
- Extent of peripheral oedema.
- Capillary refill time.
- Blood pressure (including mean arterial pressure).
- Heart rate and rhythm.
- ECG.
- Central venous pressure.
- Cardiac output monitoring.
- If the patient has had an echo, document the results and when it was performed.
- Document any cardiac medication, including inotropes, vasopressors and antihypertensive agents.

Renal system

- Average urine output (ml/hour).
- Total fluid intake and output in last 24 hours, and overall balance.
- The patient's weight (are they becoming overloaded?).
- Has the patient required diuretics in the last 24 hours?
- Have they required renal replacement therapy (i.e. dialysis or filtration) in the last 24 hours?
- Electrolyte results.

Gastrointestinal system

- Note any abnormalities on examination.
- By what route (e.g. nasogastric, TPN, none) is the patient being fed?
- What kind of feed are they receiving?
- Is it being absorbed?
- What is the rate at which feed is being given?

- When did the patient last open their bowels?
- Are they on any medication for their gastrointestinal system (e.g. prokinetics, laxatives, gastric pH-modifying drugs)?
- Note the liver function test results.

Haematology
- Haemoglobin, platelet and clotting results.
- Has the patient required transfusions in the last 24 hours?
- Are they on any anticoagulation medication?

Neurological system
- What is the patient's sedation score?
- What is their Glasgow Coma Scale score?
- Neurological examination (pupils, power tone and reflexes).
- Neurological medication (sedatives, muscle relaxants, anti-epileptics).
- If the patient is on a neurosurgical unit, document the intracranial pressure, the amount of drainage from an EVD catheter, and whether they required treatment for neurological problems overnight.

Microbiology
- Document any organisms that have been cultured and their sensitivities.
- What antibiotics is the patient taking, and for how long have they been taking these?
- Document the highest temperature in the last 24 hours.
- Document the white cell count.
- Is the patient on activated protein C?

Lines
- What lines are in place?
- How long have they been in place?
- Is the site clean?

General
- When were the patient's relatives last spoken to?
- Does the patient have treatment limitations or a 'Do not resuscitate' order?
- Have you reviewed the prescription chart and any recent investigations?

Summary of problems

- List the problems that your systemic review has highlighted.

Treatment plan

- List the jobs that need to be done.
- Finally, sign and date your record and make sure that your name is legible.

3

Face masks, continuous positive airway pressure (CPAP) and airways

Shelley Newman and Nitin Arora

Basic assessment and resuscitation of any critically ill patient follow an 'ABCDE' approach:
- **A**irway
- **B**reathing
- **C**irculation
- **D**isability
- **E**xposure.

Oxygen delivery to the lungs and bloodstream (and removal of carbon dioxide) is the ultimate aim in **A**irway and **B**reathing. To manage hypoxia appropriately you need to be aware of the various methods of delivering the correct amount of oxygen to the patient. There will be some methods with which you are familiar, and others that are more unique to the critical care environment. The choice of device will be influenced by the amount of oxygen/support required, efficacy and patient compliance.

Learning objectives

- State the advantages and disadvantages of various methods of oxygen delivery, and the main differences between them.
- Observe a patient and identify what method is being used (this is helpful for ward rounds!).
- Choose an appropriate oxygen delivery device for a hypoxic patient.
- Start to think about higher levels of respiratory support, including methods of securing the airway.

Oxygen delivery without airway/respiratory support

If the patient is maintaining their airway and breathing spontaneously, supplementary oxygen may be all that is required. Depending on the percentage of oxygen that you wish to deliver, there is a choice of masks available.

The amount of oxygen that is being provided is expressed as a percentage (%) or fraction of inspired oxygen (FiO_2), with 100% O_2 being equivalent to an FiO_2 of 1.0. Flow rates are expressed in litres per minute (l/min).

Room air delivers 21% oxygen (FiO_2 of 0.21).

Nasal cannulae

- Clear prongs that fit into each nostril, with tubing secured behind the ears and under the chin.
- Deliver 24–40% oxygen, with flow rates of 2–4 l/min; can deliver up to 6 l/min.
- Minimally disruptive, so the patient can eat, drink and talk normally.
- Only air entering through the nose is supplemented with oxygen.
- Higher flow rates can cause discomfort and bleeding.
- Cannot reliably determine how much oxygen the patient is receiving.
- Only suitable for patients with lower oxygen requirements.

Simple (Hudson) face mask

- Clear mask that fits around the mouth and nose.
- Delivers 35–60% oxygen, with flow rates of 5–10 l/min.
- Needs to be removed if the patient wants to eat or drink.
- Air is mixed with oxygen in varying ratios, so it is not possible to determine exactly how much oxygen is being delivered.

- Requires a flow rate of at least 5 l/min to wash expired carbon dioxide from the mask chamber.

Venturi face mask

- Clear mask that is attached to one of a range of coloured 'Venturi' valves with evenly spaced holes.
- These valves deliver a fixed percentage of oxygen to the mask by entraining air through different-sized holes in the valve.
- Each valve states the flow rate required and the percentage of oxygen that will be delivered to the patient.
- This is the only method that delivers an accurately measured percentage of oxygen to the patient via a simple face mask.

COLOUR OF VALVE	FLOW RATE REQUIRED (L/MIN)	OXYGEN DELIVERED (%)
Blue	2	24
White	4	28
Yellow	6	35
Red	8	40
Green	12	60

Face mask with reservoir bag

- Clear mask with one-way valves and a reservoir bag beneath.
- Delivers up to 80–98% oxygen with a flow of 15 l/min, depending on the fit of the mask and the respiratory rate of the patient.
- Some room air/expired carbon dioxide will inevitably enter the mask, but the one-way valves help to prevent this.
- Of all the face masks, this type delivers the highest percentage of oxygen.

Oxygen delivery with respiratory support

The following two methods of oxygen delivery provide extra respiratory support to the patient in the form of **continuous positive airway pressure (CPAP)** and **positive end-expiratory pressure (PEEP)**, measured in cmH_2O. A fixed amount of pressure is delivered, which helps to splint the patient's lungs and improve gas exchange. This is useful if oxygenation is low on the face mask with reservoir bag, or if the patient is tiring. The PEEP is titrated to response (clinical picture, oxygen saturation and arterial blood gas results). Patients can also be non-invasively ventilated using the mask.

CPAP mask
- Tight-fitting mask that is strapped around the head, and which fits over the mouth and nose.
- It is possible to alter the PEEP, oxygen percentage and oxygen flow rate.
- The flow of oxygen can be much greater than the rate of 15 l/min which is normally provided via facemask, due to much wider tubing, improving overall oxygen delivery even with higher respiratory rates.
- Can be claustrophobic, and is not well tolerated by some patients.
- Needs to be removed to allow the patient to eat and drink. Therefore support will be temporarily lost.

CPAP hood
- Clear hood that fits over the head and around the neck, with a strap under each arm.
- Provides the same settings as the CPAP mask.
- Can be less claustrophobic, and patients find it easier to talk while wearing this device.
- The cap on the side of the hood can be removed to allow the patient to eat and drink. However, as with removal of the mask, support will be temporarily lost.

Non-invasive positive pressure ventilation (NIPPV)
- Is also referred to as BiPAP or NIV.
- Uses the same mask as CPAP.
- Delivers two alternating levels of pressure which can both be adjusted.
- The higher pressure provides inspiratory pressure support.
- The lower pressure facilitates expiration. However, it still maintains a level of PEEP to help to prevent collapse of the lung bases.
- Useful to trial in patients who may not be suitable for intubation for various reasons.
- Used to support ventilation in patients with COPD who have type 2 respiratory failure.

- May be less well tolerated by the patient than CPAP, due to the alternating pressures.

Oxygen delivery with airway support

The following are adjuncts to secure a patent airway in the patient who tires or who has a low Glasgow Coma Scale (GCS) score. These devices are physically positioned in the airway to keep it open. They can be attached to the CPAP machine to provide the support described above, or to a ventilator.

Endotracheal tube (ETT)
- Clear flexible tube with length markings (in cm) along the side.
- Inserted orally with a laryngoscope while the patient is sedated (usually by an anaesthetist or other airway-trained health professional), and secured in position with fabric tape.
- Adult tubes have an inflatable cuff at the distal end to occlude the airway around the tube. This is inflated via a port at the proximal end.
- Available with a range of diameters, typically size 7.0 for females and size 8.0 for males.
- If the patient arrives on the unit from theatre, a chest X-ray is required to ensure adequate placement (in the trachea, past the vocal cords and above the carina).
- ETT use is associated with an increased risk of chest infection.
- The inflated cuff can cause tracheal stenosis if it is too inflated or sited for too long.
- Generally need to be changed every 10–14 days. If longer-term support is needed, a tracheostomy may be required (see below).

Tracheostomy
- Resembles a shorter, more curved endotracheal tube.
- Has an inflatable cuff.
- Can be sited on the unit (percutaneously) or in theatre (surgically).
- Used in patients who require longer-term airway support.
- Enters the airway via the anterior neck, below the thyroid cartilage and the cricothyroid membrane.
- The tube is secured by tape strapped around the neck.

- It is an invasive procedure that requires puncture/incision of the skin, the subcutaneous tissue and the anterior wall of the trachea.
- It will take time to heal when it has been removed, and is likely to leave a scar.
- As the tracheostomy does not pass through the vocal cords, it can be fitted with a speaking (or Passy-Muir) valve to allow the patient to 'talk past the tube.' This is a one-way valve that allows the patient to breathe in through the tube and out through their nose and mouth.

If the patient has an ETT or tracheostomy fitted, they can either be mechanically ventilated or breathe spontaneously. CPAP and PEEP can be delivered to provide the benefits described above.

4

The ventilator

Irfan Chaudry

'What settings do you want on the ventilator for this patient?'

In this chapter we shall look at the basics of why we ventilate a patient and the settings that are used. A basic knowledge of respiratory physiology and respiratory failure will be assumed. More advanced methods of ventilating patients are beyond the scope of this chapter, and the interested reader is directed to the Further reading section.

Learning objectives
- Why it is necessary to ventilate.
- How to set up the ventilator.
- Common pitfalls and complications.

Why it is necessary to ventilate
We need to ventilate patients for a number of reasons, which can be divided into two broad categories:

- **extrapulmonary:**
  — *central nervous system:* coma, overdose of sedative or narcotic medication, failure of respiratory centres
  — *neuromuscular:* myasthenia gravis, electrolyte imbalance, diaphragmatic dysfunction
  — *musculoskeletal:* trauma, flail chest.
- **pulmonary:**
  — airway obstruction, non-compliant lung tissue (e.g. pneumonia, ARDS).

For the reasons listed above we need to augment normal respiratory function, which basically involves transporting oxygen from the atmosphere into the tissues, and removing carbon dioxide from the tissues via the lungs, causing minimal damage on the way.

We shall assume that the patient has been connected to the ventilator via a closed suction device and some form of humidification.

How to set up the ventilator

The first aim of ventilation is to get oxygen into the patient:
- **PaO_2:** by altering the inspired oxygen concentration (FiO_2), the alveolar pressure and alveolar ventilation
- **ventilation/perfusion (V/Q) ratio:** by recruiting collapsed alveoli to reduce the amount of intra-pulmonary shunt this can be done using positive end-expiratory pressure (PEEP), usually 5–10 cmH_2O.

The second aim is to remove carbon dioxide from the patient. This is achieved by manipulating alveolar ventilation:

$$\text{alveolar ventilation} = \text{respiratory rate} \times (\text{tidal volume} - \text{dead space volume}).$$

The third aim is to minimise any damage caused to the pulmonary system:
- **volutrauma:** damage due to volume overload of the alveoli
- **barotrauma:** damage due to pressure overload of the alveoli.

The aim is to achieve tidal volumes of 6–8 ml/kg in non-compliant lungs (or up to 10 ml/kg in 'normal' lungs), and mean airway pressures of around 25–30 cmH_2O. Peak pressures greater than 45 cmH_2O are associated with alveolar damage (*see* Chapter 24).

The mode of ventilation is also important when setting up. The following modes are available:

- **continuous mandatory ventilation (CMV):** all respiratory movements are made by the ventilator, with no patient input
- **synchronised intermittent mandatory ventilation (SIMV):** the patient has respiratory effort and this is synchronised with ventilator-delivered breaths
- **SPONT:** a spontaneous mode in which the patient breathes on their own, usually with some form of support (e.g. pressure support).

Other modes are linked to certain manufacturers (e.g. BiLevel, BiPaP).

The next step is to decide whether ventilator breaths are to be volume controlled (VCV) or pressure controlled (PCV).

So, for example, a starting point for a 70 kg man could be as follows:

- FiO_2: 100%
- SIMV: VCV tidal volume set at 500 ml, rate set at 12 breaths/min
- PEEP: 5 cmH$_2$O.

Remember to use measured parameters (e.g. SaO_2, arterial blood gases) and clinical assessment (e.g. ascertaining whether the patient is synchronising with the ventilator) to guide further settings.

Common pitfalls and complications

As with all problems with ventilated patients, check your patient first before checking the ventilator. If the problem is with the ventilator, remember that you can isolate the patient by manual ventilation with a resuscitation bag.

- **Ventilator-associated lung injury:** this can be avoided by using protective strategies (*see* Chapter 24).
- **Barotrauma (e.g. pneumothorax, air embolism):** this can be avoided by not using excess pressures.
- **Cardiovascular compromise (due to excessive intrathoracic pressure and poor venous return):** again avoid excess pressure and PEEP.
- **Raised intracranial pressure:** again could be due to increased intrathoracic pressure or raised $PaCO_2$ (*see* Chapter 13).
- **Ventilator-associated pneumonia:** adopting an appropriate package of care may reduce the risk.

Further reading

- Bersten A, Soni N. *Oh's Intensive Care Manual*, 6th edn. Philadelphia, PA: Butterworth-Heinemann; 2009.
- Whitehead T, Slutsky AS. The pulmonary physician in critical care. 7. Ventilator-induced lung injury. *Thorax.* 2002; **57:** 635–42.
- Acute Respiratory Distress Syndrome Network. Ventilation with lower tidal volumes as compared with traditional tidal volumes for acute lung injury and the acute respiratory distress syndrome. *N Engl J Med.* 2000; **342:** 1301–8.

5

Monitoring the critical care patient

Rachel Saxon and Shondipon Laha

In critical care it is common for all aspects of monitoring to be recorded in one place (i.e. on a daily observations chart), so the different aspects of the same system (e.g. the cardiovascular system) can be compared in order to identify any trends.

Different ICUs will use different monitors, but the majority will display a combination of the following measurements: pulse, blood pressure (intermittent or continuous trace), mean arterial pressure (MAP), respiratory rate, oxygen saturations and central venous pressure. Additional monitors, such as intracranial pressure (ICP) monitors, may also be found in specialist ICUs.

The following parameters can be monitored non-invasively:

- **Pulse** can be measured by means of ECG electrodes, pulse oximeter or manually (normal range, 60–100 beats/min; bradycardia, < 60 beats/min; tachycardia, > 100 beats/min).
- **Blood pressure** is usually measured using a cuff on either the upper or lower limb. This will give intermittent readings. A continuous trace can only be achieved by invasive monitoring.
- **Mean arterial pressure (MAP)** is defined as the average pressure over a whole cardiac cycle, and can be calculated from the systolic and

diastolic values. The MAP is usually displayed in parentheses after the blood pressure.

There is no agreed normal range, but rather the target is usually to maintain adequate perfusion of the organs – for example, by using urine output as a marker of kidney (and thus other organ) perfusion.

- **Electrocardiogram (ECG) trace** is a graphical representation on a monitor of the electrical activity of the heart. If the trace appears abnormal it is worth checking the arterial line trace (if this is available) for concordant abnormal activity.
- **Respiratory rate** is either measured with the ECG electrodes or counted manually.
- **Oxygen saturation** is measured using a pulse oximeter. It provides an indication of oxygenation, not ventilation. Bear in mind that the saturations are measured with a colorimeter, so the fingernails must be free of nail varnish, and if the patient is peripherally shut down, placing a probe on the earlobe rather than the finger may give a more accurate reading.
- **Temperature** will usually be recorded hourly using a tympanic thermometer.
- **Urine output.** The vast majority of patients will be catheterised, and hourly urine output will be measured. This can then be compared with fluid input over the same time period in order to obtain an idea of the fluid balance. It is important to take into consideration insensible fluid losses that cannot be measured.

The following are examples of invasive monitoring:
- **Arterial lines** are cannulae which are sited in an artery (usually the radial artery, but the femoral, brachial and dorsalis pedis may also be used) and connected to a transducer that gives a continuous blood pressure trace. This technique also allows regular blood sampling through the arterial line.
- **Central lines** are catheters that are fed into a large 'central' vein (the femoral, internal jugular or subclavian vein) and again connected to a transducer. They give a measurement of venous blood pressure and allow administration of total parenteral nutrion, medication and fluid into a large vein. This could also be required if medication cannot be administered peripherally or if venous access is particularly difficult.

In the majority of patients, central venous pressure can be used as a reflection of right (and thus left) ventricular preload. The exceptions to this are patients with severe ventricular dysfunction or pulmonary hypertension, and those on mechanical ventilation.

- **Intracranial pressure (ICP)** is the pressure inside the cranial vault. It is measured via an ICP bolt connected to a transducer. (The normal ICP is in the range 0–10 mmHg, and a sustained increase above 20 mmHg is considered abnormal). A raised ICP is quite common when weaning patients off sedation.

There are other more specialist monitors that you may encounter in the critical care setting, such as cardiac output monitoring, which you need to be aware of but which are not described here.

6

Communication

Mark Pugh

Why is communication so important?

Good communication within the multi-disciplinary team and with patients and their relatives is essential to the efficient running of a critical care unit. In 2008, the NHS received 90 000 written complaints, of which 1 in 10 cited poor communication as the main cause for concern.

Effective communication is essential to the well-being of your patient and to your future medical career. It will be assessed on a regular basis throughout your training.

In critical care, your patient's outcome relies upon good communication within the critical care multi-disciplinary team, with the referring specialty team and with most other departments within the hospital. The majority of this communication will involve junior members of the clinical team, which means *you*.

Who will I be communicating with?

On the critical care unit

- The patient and their family/next of kin.

- The nurse who is looking after the patient.
- The sister/charge nurse with overall responsibility.
- Junior and senior medical colleagues.
- Allied healthcare professionals (physiotherapists, dietitians, pharmacists, radiographers, etc.).

In the hospital
- Referring teams, emergency department, anaesthetists.
- Other departments (e.g. laboratory staff, radiology, pharmacy).

Outside the hospital
- The patient's general practitioner.
- The coroner/police.

How can I communicate effectively within the multi-disciplinary team?

Effective communication is dependent to a large extent upon mutual respect and trust. It is essential to acknowledge everyone's role within the multi-disciplinary team, and to recognise that patient outcomes depend upon all aspects of care delivery, not just the doctors' role. Remember that **you are a small yet essential cog in a large machine.**

For some medical practitioners this is a difficult concept to grasp. Some advice for a long and hassle-free career is given below.

ALWAYS
- Introduce yourself to the patient and to the nurse who is looking after them.
- Listen to and acknowledge the concerns of others.
- Explain the reasons for your decisions.
- Admit when you don't know the answer.
- Admit when you are wrong.

NEVER
- Ignore or talk down to patients or members of the multi-disciplinary team.
- 'Blag' or work outside your proven competencies.

- Argue or disagree forcibly with team members in front of patients, relatives or other staff.
- Try to 'score points' within the team.
- Try to hide your mistakes or omissions.

For situations in which you are discussing clinical issues, especially over the telephone with senior medical staff, there is a widely used system to aid communication, namely the SBAR approach:

- **S**ituation:
  — Identify yourself and the unit you are calling from
  — Identify the patient and the reason for your call
  — Describe your concern.
- **B**ackground:
  — Give the patient's reason for and date of admission
  — Explain the significant medical history
  — Inform the doctor of the admission diagnosis/prior procedures/ medications/allergies/laboratory and diagnostic results.
- **A**ssessment:
  — Vital signs
  — Clinical impressions/concerns
  — Measures already taken.
- **R**ecommendations:
  — Explain what you need – be specific about what you need and when. For instance, 'I need you to see this patient now' rather than 'I would like you to see this patient soon'
  — Make suggestions
  — Clarify expectations, especially if advice is given over the phone – repeat it back to ensure accuracy.

This system works well, with a few provisos. Before picking up the phone, always make sure that:

- *you* know the patient and the situation well
- *you* have carried out a thorough assessment, including examining the patient
- *you* have started simple measures to improve the situation and asked for appropriate help within the multi-disciplinary team
- *you* have a clear idea of what *you* want to happen.

As with all communication, a concise account of the conversation should be entered in the notes. The recommendations/actions to be taken should be clearly stated. The account should be dated, a time should be entered (using the 24-hour clock), and a legible signature should be provided, with your name and position printed clearly underneath. Remember to record who you spoke to – the notes remain a legal document and are your best defence should matters be challenged at a later date.

How can I communicate effectively with patients and relatives?

Not all patients in critical care are unconscious.

ALWAYS
- Introduce yourself to the patient as though they can hear you (they often can, despite appearances).
- Explain what you are about to do before performing an examination or procedure.
- Treat the patient with respect and dignity.
- Be positive.

NEVER
- Assume that the patient is unconscious.
- Make comments about the patient's prognosis or progress (unless they are positive) within earshot.
- Make disparaging or hurtful comments.
- Gossip or talk about other patients within earshot.

When major decisions about treatment are made, remember to involve the patient directly wherever possible. A lack of capacity does not mean that you should not attempt to explain what is happening and why.

How do I break bad news?

Most UK doctors now undergo extensive training as undergraduates in communication skills, including how to break bad news. However, this does not make you an expert.

Ideally, the most senior clinician available should lead conversations about withdrawing and withholding treatment, preferably in the daytime when there is plenty of support for patients and their relatives immediately available.

Whenever the opportunity arises, watch others breaking bad news. You will see both good and bad ways of going about it, and be able to decide for yourself what works for you in this situation. When breaking bad news for the first time, always take someone more senior with you for moral support.

By far the best model approach for breaking bad news was described by Buckman, and although primarily designed for use by oncologists, it is easily adaptable to critical care. The approach is summarised below.

SPIKES model
- **S**etting, listening skills
- **P**atient's/relatives' perceptions
- **I**nvite patient/relative to share information
- **K**nowledge transmission
- **E**xplore emotions and empathise
- **S**ummarise and strategise

Remember that in the case of conscious patients you should always attempt to talk with the patient first. Some patients may not wish to discuss major issues, but you should always attempt to do so, and document that you have. Before speaking to the relatives of a conscious patient, first ensure that the patient is happy for you to do so.

The setting is important. Every unit should have an interview room of sufficient size to allow these conversations to occur away from the bedside and in privacy.

The model works well because it ensures that the majority of the process is concentrated on *you listening* to the patient's or relative's perceptions and fears, rather than being focused on the doctor giving information and/or making decisions.

Some more advice for an easy life is given below.

ALWAYS
- Ensure that you know the patient and their diagnosis and prognosis well.

- Take the nurse who is looking after the patient with you.
- Introduce yourself and any other members of the team who are present, and ask the family members to introduce themselves (I have mistaken a patient's wife for their mother, and vice versa).
- Establish the patient's known wishes.
- Keep matters simple, and avoid the use of jargon.
- Take your time. If a family is struggling to understand and come to terms with what you are saying, back off and arrange to speak to them again later.
- Use clear terms (e.g. 'die', 'futile').
- Document clearly the outcome of the meeting.

NEVER

- Begin a conversation without full knowledge of the situation.
- Rush.
- Be ambiguous.
- Blame other teams or specialties for a poor outcome.
- Break a patient confidence.

Conclusion

Effective communication can be easily achieved if you remember to respect and value those around you. Remember to treat people as you would wish to be treated yourself and you won't go far wrong.

Further reading

- Information Centre for Health and Social Care. *Data on Written Complaints in the NHS 2008–2009*. Leeds: Information Centre for Health and Social Care; 2009.
- NHS Institute for Innovation and Improvement. *Safer Care. SBAR – Situation-Background-Assessment-Recommendation*. Warwick: NHS Institute for Innovation and Improvement; 2010.
- Buckman R. *How to Break Bad News: a guide for health care professionals*. Baltimore, MD: Johns Hopkins University Press; 1992.

7

Capacity and consent

Michael Stewart and Nitin Arora

Introduction

In order to understand the importance of consent (and the capacity to give consent) it is necessary to understand the legal definitions of battery and assault.

- Battery is the unlawful application of physical force to another.
- Assault is an attempt to commit battery or an act that may reasonably cause fear of imminent battery.

Therefore, unless we have permission to touch the patient, many of the interventions that we perform are illegal.

Consent

Physical contact and medical interventions do not constitute battery if the patient has given consent for them to be carried out. There are three main forms of consent that are applicable.

- **Implied consent:** the patient makes an action to facilitate a proposed intervention (e.g. they hold an arm out when asked for a blood sample).

- **Explicit consent:** an intervention is discussed with the patient, and they agree to have it performed (e.g. they sign a consent form for a laparotomy). The agreement may be verbal or in writing, and there is no legal difference in the validity of these. However, it is easier to prove that the patient gave consent if it is in writing.
- **Presumed consent:** in a patient who cannot consent (if they lack capacity), this is an assumption that they would agree to the intervention if they did have capacity. Presumed consent applies if the intervention is considered to be in the patient's best interest, and there is no indication that they would have refused if they had capacity.

Implied and explicit consent are only valid if the patient has capacity, whereas presumed consent only applies if the patient lacks capacity.

Legally, a patient with capacity can agree to or refuse any treatment that is offered. They do not, in law, have the right to demand a treatment that is considered inappropriate or futile by the clinician who is caring for them. However, it is considered best practice to seek a second consultant's opinion before refusing an intervention that the patient requests.

Consent is the legal agreement to an intervention. Assent is an agreement given by someone who cannot formally consent. This could be the patient if they lack capacity (e.g. a young child can agree to a blood test that a parent has formally given consent for), or the next of kin (e.g. agreeing to an operation where presumed consent has given the legal authority to proceed).

Capacity

To be able to give valid consent, a patient must be competent to do so. Competence is defined as having capacity, as judged by meeting the following criteria:

1 understanding and believing the information that is given
2 retaining the information
3 weighing up the information in order to reach a balanced decision
4 communicating that decision.

The decision must be considered, but need not appear sensible to those hearing it. In practice, it can be very difficult to differentiate between a rational decision made by someone with different values to oneself, and an irrational decision. If there is any doubt, a second opinion is always recommended. In a non-emergency situation, this may occasionally require a legal ruling.

Capacity should be judged against the severity of the decision that is being made, and is not 'all or nothing.' A person may well be competent to decide whether or not they want an analgesic, but lack capacity to agree to major cardiac surgery. One of the principles of the Mental Capacity Act 2005 is that patients should be supported to make as many of their own decisions as possible.

Lack of capacity

If a patient has previously had capacity, there are two principal ways in which they can arrange to consent to decisions made when they lack capacity:

- An advance directive is a legal document that was completed, signed and witnessed by the patient while they had capacity, setting out the interventions to which they would and would not consent. This has the same force as their own decision, so long as it is genuine and covers the situation that has arisen. Verifying this may be difficult in the emergency situation.
- A person with power of attorney is an individual who was appointed by the patient while they had capacity, whom they have given authority to consent to or refuse treatment on their behalf. Again, decisions made by the attorney should be treated identically to decisions made by the patient.

In the absence of power of attorney or an advance directive, the treatment of a patient who lacks capacity should be to provide what is felt to be in their best interest. The final decision on this is usually made by the medical team that is caring for the patient, but with due regard for the previously expressed opinions of the patient.

Determining what is in the patient's best interest should involve discussion with someone representing the view of the patient. The Mental Capacity Act 2005 sets out an order of preference, which includes the patient, relatives, friends and long-term carers. If it is impossible to contact any of these individuals, an Independent Mental Capacity Advocate (IMCA) should be appointed.

The role of the relative, friend, carer or IMCA is to represent the views that the patient has previously expressed. They are asked to set aside their own opinions as much as they can.

If there is a significant disagreement about what is in the best interest of the patient, the Court of Protection (established by the Mental Capacity Act 2005) can be asked for a ruling.

Children

The law relating to children is more complex. The basic principles are as follows.

- Children aged 16–17 years.
  - In Scotland, the legal age of capacity is 16. In other UK jurisdictions, a person who has attained the age of 16 is assumed to have the same capacity as an adult to consent to treatment.
  - Information about these patients should not be revealed to their parents without their consent.
- Children under 16 years.
  - A child under the age of 16 years may have capacity. The legal test is for 'Gillick competence' – they are deemed to be Gillick competent if they can understand the implications of the decision that they are making. This competence may depend on the age and maturity of the child and the complexity of the procedure to be undertaken.
  - In general it is best practice to also obtain parental assent, but if a Gillick competent child insists on confidentiality, this must be respected.
  - A person with parental responsibility can always consent for a child under 16 years of age, even if the child is Gillick competent.
- Withholding consent.
  - If the child is not Gillick competent, the parents can consent on behalf of the child, even if the child is refusing the treatment. However, doctors must decide whether overriding the child's refusal of consent is in their best interest.
  - Patients aged 16–17 can withhold consent to treatment, but this can be overruled (except in Scotland) in exceptional circumstances if it is considered to be in their best interests, either by someone with parental responsibility or by the courts.

- Treatment in emergencies.
  - In an emergency situation, when a person with parental responsibility is not available to consent for treatment, the doctor has to consider what is in the child's best interest and act accordingly. This should be discussed with a senior medical colleague and documented fully.

In all cases that are not clear cut, senior medical advice must be sought at an early stage and, sometimes, legal advice may also be needed.

Mental Health Act 1983

The Mental Health Act 1983 sets out situations in which a patient may be detained for assessment and treatment of mental health disorders, without their consent. No part of the act permits treatment for physical disorders without the usual process of consent. The fact that a patient is detained under a section of the act does not make it legal to treat a physical ailment without the patient's consent.

However, the underlying mental health problem may mean that the patient is unable to weigh up the information provided as required in order to have capacity, and therefore cannot consent to or refuse treatment. In this situation, it may be necessary to treat them with the presumed consent that is allowed for in common law, as discussed earlier.

Further reading

- Department of Health. *Mental Health Act 1983*. London: Department of Health; 1983.
- General Medical Council. *0–18 Years: guidance for all doctors*. London: General Medical Council; 2007. www.gmc-uk.org/static/documents/content/GMC_0-18_0911.pdf (accessed 25 July 2010).
- Medical Protection Society. *Factsheet. Consent – children and young people*. London: Medical Protection Society; 2010. www.medicalprotection.org/uk/factsheets/consent-children (accessed 25 July 2010).
- Office of Public Sector Information. *Mental Capacity Act 2005*. London: Office of Public Sector Information; 2005.

8

Analgesia, sedation and muscle relaxation

Steven Benington

The intensive care unit is an uncomfortable place for patients, who are subjected to many painful and distressing procedures. Simply tolerating an endotracheal tube can be a traumatic experience. Repeated insertion of intravenous lines, chest suction, changes of position and other interventions engender further discomfort. In addition, many surgical patients have post-operative pain to contend with. Adequate analgesia and anxiolysis are therefore key components of the management of these patients.

General principles
- Most analgesic and sedative agents are given as continuous intravenous infusions titrated to patient response.
- When the rate of a sedative or analgesic infusion is *increased*, the length of time required for this change to take full effect is around five times the half-life of the drug. Morphine has a long half-life, of about 3 hours. Increasing the infusion rate alone would therefore take around 15 hours to reach full effect. To avoid this problem, a **bolus dose** of the drug should be given as a 'top-up' when increasing the rate.

- Similarly, when the rate of infusion is *decreased*, the length of time required for this change to take full effect is often prolonged. For this reason, the infusion should be stopped completely to minimise the time required for the effects of the drug to wear off, and it can then be restarted at a lower rate when the patient is more alert.
- For most analgesic and sedative drugs, the longer the infusion has been running, the longer the offset when it is discontinued. This is because a 'reservoir' of drug builds up in the patient's tissues over time, which maintains blood (and brain) levels of the drug. A midazolam infusion that has been running for a week may take several days to wear off when stopped. This problem can be minimised by the use of a daily **sedation hold**.

Analgesia

Almost all ICU patients require some form of analgesia. In a minority of cases this will be limited to simple analgesics, such as paracetamol. This can be given either enterally if the patient has a functioning gastrointestinal tract, or intravenously. The intravenous form reaches the tissues in higher concentrations and is more effective.

Non-steroidal anti-inflammatory drugs (NSAIDs) are infrequently used in the critical care setting, due to the increased risk of acute renal dysfunction and gastrointestinal haemorrhage in this setting. However, certain patients may benefit (e.g. young fit trauma patients with painful injuries).

Regional anaesthetic techniques are useful for numbing a painful area, thereby reducing the need for polypharmacy. A correctly sited epidural can eliminate the need for morphine following a laparotomy, and a femoral nerve block can eliminate the pain of a fractured femoral shaft. Any healthcare professional who is administering local or regional anaesthesia should be aware of the maximum toxic dose of local anaesthetic and the contraindications to such techniques. Unfortunately, most ICU patients have pain and discomfort from many areas, which limits the usefulness of such techniques.

Opioids are the mainstay of ICU analgesia, and are usually given by intravenous infusion. Commonly used drugs include morphine, fentanyl, alfentanil and remifentanil. As well as providing analgesia, these drugs provide a degree of sedation.

Each ICU will have a particular standard concentration and dosing range (e.g. fentanyl 50 mcg/ml run at a rate of 1–10 ml/hour).

The commonly used opioids are compared in Table 8.1. The dosing information that is provided (concentration of infusion/diluents/infusion rate) is intended only as a guide; each ICU may have a slightly different 'recipe.'

TABLE 8.1 Opioids used on the ICU

DRUG	DOSING INFORMATION	ADVANTAGES	DISADVANTAGES
Morphine	1 mg/ml N saline 1–10 ml/hour	Cheap. High level of familiarity with its use. Reliable analgesia	Long half-life, so takes many hours for effect to wear off when stopped. Relatively slow onset (30 minutes for a bolus dose to reach peak effect)
Fentanyl	50 µg/ml N saline 1–10 ml/hour	More rapid onset than morphine	Can still accumulate in the tissues, so offset time increases in proportion to duration of infusion
Alfentanil	500 µg/ml N saline 1–10 ml/hour	Near-instant onset. Rapid offset if short-duration infusion	
Remifentanil	100 µg/ml N saline 1–10 ml/hour	Ultra-short-acting. Effect wears off in minutes even when infused for days, due to metabolism in the blood	Relatively expensive. Potent respiratory depressant. Not suitable for bolus dosing

These drugs must be titrated to effect, since patients will respond differently depending on their height, weight, renal and liver function, and many other factors. Patients with renal failure are particularly sensitive to morphine, which has an active metabolite that is normally excreted in the urine, but accumulates in renal impairment. When titrating opioids to effect, consider the following:

- Does the patient appear to be in pain (e.g. grimacing, restless, sweaty)?
- Do the observations (blood pressure, heart rate) suggest pain?
- In conscious patients, how severe is the pain on a scale of 1 to 10?

Sedation

Opioids have a sedating effect, and a large number of patients may be managed without formal sedatives (also known as hypnotics and anxiolytics).

However, many patients require deeper sedation to facilitate painful procedures or cooperation with ventilation, or to rest the brain in cases of neurological injury. The most widely used agents are propofol and midazolam. As with opioids, sedatives have a standard concentration on a given ICU, and generally are titrated to effect in the range of 1–20 ml/hour (*see* Table 8.2).

TABLE 8.2 Sedative agents on the ICU

DRUG	DOSING INFORMATION	ADVANTAGES	DISADVANTAGES
Propofol	1% (10 mg/ml) Neat 1–30 ml/hour OR 2% (20 mg/ml) Neat 1–20 ml/hour	Potent anaesthetic, sedative in smaller doses. Rapid effect. Reliably 'flattens' the combative patient. Easily titratable. Relatively quick offset even after prolonged infusion	Causes hypotension in larger doses. Potent respiratory depressant. Can cause metabolic acidosis/cardiac failure if used at high doses for prolonged periods. May cause hyperlipidaemia and deranged liver function tests
Midazolam	1 mg/ml Normal saline 1–20 ml/hour	A benzodiazepine. Causes less hypotension than propofol. Excellent anxiolytic properties	Slow offset when used for prolonged periods of time. Accumulates in renal failure
Clonidine	15 µg/ml Normal saline 1–5 ml/hour	α-2 adrenoceptor agonist. Sedates with little respiratory depression. Low incidence of delirium. Useful in alcohol withdrawal	Can cause hypotension and bradycardia. Slower onset; less useful for immediate sedation of the dangerously agitated patient
Thiopentone	25 mg/ml Sterile water 20–50 ml/hour	A barbiturate. Potent anticonvulsant. Lowers intracranial pressure. Mainly used in neurosurgical patients	Very long offset time after prolonged infusion

Sedative drugs are titrated to effect following the general principles outlined above. Most sedatives have no analgesic properties, and opioids should generally be given as well. Various scoring systems are available to assess the patient's level of sedation. Generally the goal is to have the patient awake and calm, unless there are specific reasons for deep sedation, such as head injury management. The decision to sedate a patient should not be taken automatically, as sedation in the ICU is associated with future psychiatric problems, including anxiety and post-traumatic stress disorder.

Daily sedation holds

For the reasons described above, the longer the infusion has been running the longer it takes for the effect to wear off. This means that ventilated patients who are otherwise ready to be extubated may stay on the ventilator many days longer than necessary because they are too sedated to breathe adequately. This wastes ICU resources and increases the patient's risk of developing ventilator-associated pneumonia. Patients may also receive unnecessary investigations such as CT scans of the brain to determine whether their slow wake-up is due to sedation or an intracranial event such as a stroke.

A daily sedation hold, where all sedation is stopped each day to allow the excess to 'wash out' of the patient, has been shown to reduce the time spent on the ventilator, as the patient is lightly sedated, cooperative and considered ready for weaning and extubation at an earlier stage.

ICU delirium

Patients on the ICU have a high incidence of delirium. In a minority of cases this is easy to spot, with the agitated patient pulling at lines and tubes. In most cases, however, delirium is of a withdrawn form that may go unrecognised. There is growing evidence to suggest that ICU delirium is an independent risk factor for mortality at 6 months. Delirium increases in proportion to the length and depth of sedation, which should therefore be kept to the minimum required for patient cooperation and safety.

Muscle relaxation

Most ICU patients do not require muscle relaxants. These drugs block neurotransmission at the neuromuscular junction, paralysing the patient. This may be desirable to facilitate mechanical ventilation if high levels of support are required or if the patient is 'fighting the ventilator.' It is also use-ful if the patient is being transferred (e.g. into the CT scanner), to prevent reflex coughing and endotracheal tube dislodgement with movement. Prolonged muscle relaxation has many serious adverse effects, including the following:

- critical illness polyneuromyopathy, causing profound weakness
- loss of diaphragmatic and intercostal muscle mass, making weaning from the ventilator difficult
- loss of protective airway reflexes, risking aspiration pneumonia and removing the ability to cough and clear secretions from the chest
- inability to assess the patient's neurological status
- risk of awareness if the patient is paralysed but inadequately sedated.

Suxamethonium

This is a 'depolarising' muscle relaxant, which means that it first causes muscle fasciculation and then paralysis for a few minutes. It is used for the emergency intubation of patients because of its quick onset (minimising the risk of aspiration) and quick offset (spontaneous breathing resumes more rapidly if difficulty in intubation and ventilation is encountered). However, it has many side-effects, including muscle pains and hyperkalaemia, and it has a relatively high incidence of anaphylaxis. It should be avoided in hyper-kalaemic patients, those with significant burns after the first 24 hours, and patients with neuromuscular disorders. In such patients suxamethonium can cause massive potassium release and cardiac arrest.

Atracurium

This is a 'non-depolarising' muscle relaxant which can be given as a bolus or infusion. It causes paralysis within 3 minutes of a bolus dose, which lasts for around 30 minutes, and may cause histamine release and bronchospasm in susceptible patients.

Ideally, patients who are receiving muscle relaxants should be monitored with a **nerve stimulator**. This is a device that passes an electric current through a peripheral nerve (commonly the ulnar nerve), causing twitching of the innervated muscles. If there is no twitching this means that there is profound muscle relaxation. **The patient must also be assessed for depth of sedation to ensure that they are not 'aware.'** Clues that the patient may be inadequately sedated include tachycardia, hypertension, mydriasis and the presence of tears.

Further reading

- Sessler CN, Varney K. Patient-focused sedation and analgesia in the ICU. *Chest*. 2008; **133:** 552–65.
- Girard TD, Pandharipande PP, Ely EW. Delirium in the intensive care unit. *Crit Care*. 2008; **12(Suppl. 3):** S3.

Drugs that work on the heart

Andrew Haughton

In this chapter we shall look at some of the medicines which can affect the cardiovascular system. We will not cover the anti-dysrhythmic drugs, as these will be discussed in a later chapter. Rather this chapter will focus on drugs that affect blood pressure. In the intensive care setting specific anti-anginal medication is rarely used for long-term management. However, GTN spray can be given under the tongue, as would be done on the ward, for patients with acute angina.

Blood pressure

In general terms we may need to either increase or decrease a patient's blood pressure. It is important to remember during this chapter that although the drug's effects are exerted on blood pressure, it is more often the flow to organs that is our primary concern. In this respect, remember always to monitor the patient holistically, and avoid merely chasing the 'perfect' blood pressure number.

First we need to consider what factors influence blood pressure. In simple terms, the heart is a pump which can vary its rate and strength of contraction. The blood is being pumped around a circulation that essentially consists of three parts. There is an arterial system in which the pressure determines the supply pressure to organs. The pressure here also influences how much the heart empties during each contraction. After this there is a capillary system, which is large and low pressure, in which flow through individual organs is therefore governed by the feeding pressure. Finally, there is a venous system which is large, and in which the pressure determines the rate of flow back to the heart.

$$\text{Heart rate} \times \text{stroke volume} = \text{cardiac output}$$

and cardiac output is proportional to blood pressure.

Increasing blood pressure

From the previous discussion it can be seen that we can increase blood pressure by increasing heart rate or by increasing stroke volume (so long as increasing one does not decrease the other at the same time!).

What is perhaps less obvious is that we can also increase blood pressure by increasing vascular tone – that is, by decreasing the arterial volume. This of course has the potential disadvantage that by increasing tone and therefore also blood pressure, we actually reduce flow (i.e. cardiac output).

If you are finding all of this a little confusing, you are not alone! At any time we rarely have accurate measures of all of these variables, and this is why it is important to remember that blood pressure alone should not be a target. If in doubt, assess whether the patient is getting better or worse in other ways (e.g. by using urine output or lactate levels as markers of perfusion).

The discussion of the drugs which follows will describe the general principles of their actions, but in individual patients the responses will vary depending on their underlying physiology. So whenever you initiate treatment with any of these drugs, consider carefully what you want to achieve. Then assess the patient response and be prepared to be wrong and to have to change the drug!

To help to categorise different medication actions, the following terms are useful:

- *inotrope* – a substance that increases cardiac muscle contraction (in almost all cases by increasing cardiac intracellular calcium levels)
- *chronotrope* – a substance that affects heart rate
- *vasopressor* – a substance that increases vascular tone and resistance

- *adrenaline* – the 'real-thing' beta agonist. It is a naturally occurring catecholamine which has a potent effect on beta receptors 1 and 2 in all areas. As such, it is a positive inotrope with a mixed effect on vascular tone depending on the tissues
- *noradrenaline* – another naturally occurring catecholamine, which is active at alpha receptors. It causes intense vasoconstriction in most arterioles, and has some moderate inotropic actions
- *dopamine* – a catecholamine precursor of the above which has some properties of both. It also works on specific dopamine receptors which cause splanchnic vasodilatation and diuresis. Its effects at alpha and beta receptors are partly dose dependent, with the beta effect predominating at low doses and the alpha effect at higher doses
- *dobutamine* – a synthetic catecholamine which is used mainly as an inotrope. It also has significant chronotropic effects
- *digoxin* – although usually now used for rate control in atrial fibrillation, in the past it was used as a treatment for heart failure. This was because of its inotropic actions, which are due to its influence at sodium potassium channels, rather than to any beta-agonist effects
- *glucagon* – primarily causes an increase in blood sugar levels, but it also has inotropic effects which are independent of beta receptors. This makes it a useful drug in cases of beta-blocker overdose
- *phosphodiesterase inhibitors* – by reducing the breakdown of cAMP, these drugs help to increase calcium levels within cells, and thus in the heart they act as inotropes. They have a broad spectrum of effects, depending on which type of enzymes they tend to inhibit. Theophylline is mainly a bronchodilator, whereas enoximone and milnirone are mainly cardiac inotropes. However, all will have an element of action in all phophodiesterase enzyme subsets
- *levosimendan* – not yet licensed in the UK, but widely used in other countries, it is unique as an inotrope in that it does not rely on increasing calcium levels within the myocardium as its final mechanism of action. Rather it increases the sensitivity to calcium, and it also has some coronary vasodilating effects.

Decreasing blood pressure

This is mainly achieved by vasodilatation and slowing of the heart rate. Hypertension is a less common problem in critical care than is hypotension, and unless the blood pressure is very high it is probably best ignored in the short term in unstable patients. It is also worth remembering that the experience of being a patient in critical care can be painful and stressful, so always consider the need for anxiolytics and analgesics when assessing a hypertensive patient.

- *Glyceryl trinitrate (GTN)*. This is a vasodilator which in low doses affects mainly veins, and at higher doses also affects arterioles. It lowers blood pressure and leaves cardiac output unaltered or moderately reduced.
- *Hydralazine*. This is an arteriolar vasodilator which lowers vascular resistance and therefore decreases blood pressure, but which can cause a reflex tachycardia.
- *Labetalol*. This is a beta and alpha blocker, so at the same time as reducing vascular resistance it also blocks any reflex tachycardia. Therefore it will reduce blood pressure and cardiac output simultaneously.
- *Phentolamine*. This is an alpha 1 and 2 blocker, so it causes vasodilation and some inotropic effects. It reduces the blood pressure with an increased cardiac output.

Practical uses

First, always ensure adequate filling pressures, perhaps by assessing the effects of a fluid bolus. In a hypertensive patient, assess the need for anxiolytics or analgesia. Always make sure that the reading is accurate. If this is an invasive blood pressure reading, check whether the transducers are at the correct level, whether it has been zeroed, and whether it is a good arterial wave form.

Generally, invasive blood pressure monitoring is needed to enable real-time titration of inotrope/vasopressor infusions.

The following are examples of typical doses and dilutions in our unit.

- *In a septic, vasodilated patient:* noradrenaline – 4 mg made up to 40 ml with 5% glucose started at 5 ml/hour and titrated up or down against response.
- *In a patient with a reduced cardiac output:* dobutamine, 250 mg made up to 50 ml with normal saline, started at 5 ml/ hour and titrated up or down according to response. If the response to dobutamine is not

adequate, consider adrenaline, 5 mg made up to 50 ml with normal saline, started at 5 ml/hour and titrated up or down.

- *In a hypotensive patient after beta-blocker overdose:* consider glucagon, 20 mg made up to 40 ml with 5% glucose, infused at 0–20 ml/hour according to response.
- *In a hypertensive patient, with normal or high heart rate:* consider labetalol, which is available as 100 mg in 20 ml, given neat at a rate of 5–30 ml/hour according to response.
- *In a hypertensive patient in whom beta blockers are contraindicated:* glyceryl trinitrate (GTN), premixed at 1 mg/ml, given at a rate of 1–20 ml/hour.

10

Nutrition and fluids

Benjamin Slater

Nutrition is easily overlooked in the daily review of critically ill patients, but is crucial to their ability to survive acute illness. The multi-disciplinary team, including dietitians, nurses and doctors, should be involved. A dietary history on admission to hospital, taken from the patient, next of kin or carers, is invaluable.

Malnutrition is common in the critically ill, and leads to reduced muscle bulk and power. This impairs respiratory and cardiac function. Malnutrition also causes immune dysfunction, anaemia, gut mucosal atrophy, poor wound healing, reduced cognitive function, depression and poor sleep pattern.

Evidence does exist for early nutritional support in critically ill trauma and burns patients. The Intensive Care National Audit and Research Council (ICNARC) is currently investigating the role of early parenteral feeding by comparison with enteral feeding in ICU patients.

It is generally accepted that oral feeding is preferable, in order to avoid the bypassing of innate gastrointestinal reflexes which naturally facilitate digestion and the absorption of nutrients. However, swallowing is often inadequate in critically ill patients, in which case enteral feeding should be commenced. This does require intact gastrointestinal function, which may be impaired in the presence of obstruction, small bowel fistula, radiation enteritis, malabsorption or intractable diarrhoea. In these circumstances, parenteral nutrition may be totally or partially indicated.

Enteral feeding can be provided by nasogastric, post-pyloric, nasojejunal or percutaneous gastrostomy tube. Post-pyloric feeding is favoured in those individuals with gastroparesis, and may be provided by weighted or 'hooked' (Tiger) tubes, with radiological confirmation of placement.

Parenteral feeding can be provided temporarily (for up to 14 days) with simple peripheral venous cannulae, but long-term feeding requires a peripherally inserted central catheter (PICC) or a tunnelled subclavian venous catheter.

Patients who are **not** severely ill or injured, and who are not at risk of refeeding problems, have the following approximate requirements:

- total energy: 25–35 kcal/kg/day
- glucose: 2 g/kg
- fat: 2 g/kg
- protein: 0.8–1.5 g/kg (0.13–0.24 g nitrogen/kg/day)
- fluid (water): 30–35 ml kg/day, or 100 ml/kg for first 10 kg, 50 ml/kg for next 10 kg, and 20 ml/kg for each kg thereafter per 24 hours
- sodium: 1–2 mmol/kg/day
- potassium: 0.7–1.0 mmol/kg/day
- magnesium and calcium: 0.1 mmol/kg/day
- phosphate: 0.2 mmol/kg/day
- vitamins: vitamins C, A, D, E and K, thiamine, riboflavin, niacin, pyridoxine and folate
- trace elements: iron, copper, manganese, zinc, iodide and fluoride.

Seriously ill or injured patients

Remember to introduce enteral or parenteral nutrition cautiously in seriously ill or injured patients.

Start at no more than 50% of the estimated target energy and protein needs, and build up to meet the full needs over the first 24–48 hours. Provide the full requirements of fluid, electrolytes, vitamins and minerals from the outset.

Calculation of energy requirements using the Schofield equation
1 Calculate the **basal metabolic rate (BMR)** using the following formula:
   - admission weight (kg) × factor + factor (depends on age and gender; consult tables).
2 Add stress factor (e.g. multiple trauma/severe sepsis, +30%).
3 Add activity factor (e.g. bed bound, +10%; mobile, +25%).
4 Add reductions (e.g. on ventilator, −15%).

This gives the total energy requirements (in kcal) per 24 hours.

Nitrogen loss can be calculated to address the required intake, but such estimates are notoriously inaccurate in critically ill patients:

$$\text{24-hour nitrogen loss (g)} = (\text{urinary urea (mmol/24 hour)} - 1 \times 0.028) + 4.0028.$$

Approximately 4 g are lost per day in faeces, skin, hair and urine as non-urea nitrogen.

Refeeding problems

Patients who have eaten little or nothing for more than 5 days should have nutrition support introduced at less than 50% of their requirements for the first 2 days. Then increase the feeding rates to meet their full needs if clinical and biochemical monitoring reveals no refeeding problems.

There is a high risk of developing refeeding problems if **one or more** of the following are present:
- BMI < 16 kg/m^2
- unintentional weight loss > 15% within the last 3–6 months
- little or no nutritional intake for > 10 days
- low levels of potassium, phosphate or magnesium prior to feeding

or if two or more of the following are present:
- BMI < 18.5 kg/m^2
- unintentional weight loss > 10% within the last 3–6 months
- little or no nutritional intake for > 5 days
- a history of alcohol abuse or of drugs, including insulin, chemotherapy, antacids and diuretics.

When prescribing for patients at high risk of developing refeeding problems, consider the following:

- starting nutrition support at a maximum of 10 kcal/kg/day, and increasing the levels slowly to meet or exceed full needs by 4–7 days
- using only 5 kcal/kg/day in **extreme** cases
- restoring circulatory volume and monitoring fluid balance and overall clinical status closely
- providing the following immediately before and during the first **10** days of feeding:
    - oral thiamine, 200–300 mg daily
    - vitamin B Co strong 1 or 2 tablets, three times daily (or full dose daily intravenous vitamin B preparation, if necessary)
    - balanced multivitamin/trace element supplement, once daily
    - potassium, 2–4 mmol/kg/day
    - phosphate, 0.3–0.6 mmol/kg/day
    - magnesium, 0.2–0.4 mmol/kg/day.
- monitoring weight daily initially, then weekly
- measuring body mass index (BMI)/triceps skin fold thickness/mid-arm circumference at least monthly.

Monitoring nutrition in the ICU
Blood tests

- Plasma sodium, potasssium, urea, creatinine, magnesium, calcium, albumin, LFTs, glucose and phosphate.
- Full blood count and mean cell volume, looking for macrocytosis (MCV > 110 fl), which is associated with vitamin B_{12} and/or folate deficiency.
- Zinc and copper deficiency – most at risk when anabolic.
- Selenium deficiency is common after left hemicolectomy. Long-term status is more accurately assessed by glutathione peroxidase.
- Iron deficiency is common with long-term parenteral feeding (reduced Fe and raised ferritin levels).
- Serum folate/vitamin B_{12}.
- Avoid excessive manganese in patients with liver disease (red blood cell count or whole blood provide a more accurate measure than serum).
- 1,25-dihydroxyvitamin D3 – requires functional kidney.

Screen patients

- Screen on admission and weekly thereafter.
- Clinical suspicion should be raised if there is unintentional weight loss, fragile skin, poor wound healing, apathy, wasted muscles, poor appetite, altered taste and sensation, impaired swallowing, altered bowel habit, loose-fitting clothing, or prolonged intercurrent illness.
- Malnourished patients:
  - BMI $< 18.5 \, \text{kg/m}^2$
  - unintentional weight loss $> 15\,\%$ in the last 3–6 months
  - BMI $< 20 \, \text{kg/m}^2$ and unintentional weight loss $> 5\%$ in the last 3–6 months.
- At risk:
  - poor absorptive capacity
  - not having eaten for the last 5 days; will not be eating for the next 5 days
  - high nutrient losses/requirements/catabolic.
- Ask the following questions:
  - Is it safe for the patient to swallow? Do they have dysphagia?
  - If it is safe, provide oral feed.
  - In malnourished/at-risk patients, in whom oral intake would be inadequate or unsafe, but who have a functional and accessible gastrointestinal tract, consider enteral tube feeding/post-pyloric feeding/duodenal/jejunal feed.
  - If more than 4 weeks of feeding are required, consider a percutaneous gastrostomy (PEG). This can be used 4 hours after insertion.

Nasogastric tube placement

- pH test < 5.5 (National Patient Safety Agency, 2005) with or without chest X-ray if a radio-opaque tube is used.
- Monitor for tube nasal erosion, blockage or fixation.
- Deliver enteral feed continuously over a period of 16–24 hours.
- If an insulin infusion is running, feed continuously if possible to avoid hypoglycaemia. Use motility agents if there is delayed gastric emptying (e.g. IV metoclopramide, erythromycin), and assess for high residual gastric volumes. Consider post-pyloric feeding.

- If the patient is constipated, use laxatives (e.g. senna, lactulose) to improve gut transit time.
- In malnourished/at-risk patients, in whom oral intake would be inadequate or unsafe, and who have a non-functional, leaking or perforated GI tract, consider total parenteral nutrition (TPN).
- Give peripheral TPN if required for less than 14 days. Pay attention to pH, tonicity and compatibility.
- If TPD is required for more than 30 days, a tunnelled subclavian central venous catheter will be needed.
- Delivery should be continuous. If it is required for more than 14 days, consider a gradual change from continuous to cyclical delivery.
- TPN is introduced at less than 50% of needs over the initial 24–48 hours.
- Micronutrients and trace elements are added.
- Stop when there is adequate enteral/oral intake.

Summary of nutritional assessment

Energy, protein, fluid, electrolyte, mineral, micronutrient and fibre needs

- Consider activity levels and the underlying clinical condition (catabolism, pyrexia, gastrointestinal tolerance, potential metabolic instability, and risk of refeeding problems).
- Consider the likely duration of nutrition support.

Intravenous fluids

It is important to remember that fluid need not be administered intravenously, and may be administered via the nasogastric tube as water.

Intravenous fluids are generally administered as compound sodium lactate (Hartmann's solution), which is a 'balanced' salt crystalloid solution with similar concentrations of salts and tonicity to body plasma. 'Normal saline' or 0.9% sodium chloride (NaCl) contains excessive sodium and chloride (154 mmol/l) compared with body plasma, and may cause hyperchloraemic acidosis. Dextrose-containing solutions have the advantage of providing glucose, but are hypotonic and are rapidly distributed beyond the extracellular fluid space.

Colloids are generally used to resuscitate the intravascular compartment in hypotension. Traditional modified gelatins (e.g. Gelofusine) and starches have a longer intravascular half-life than crystalloids (3–12 hours vs. 20 minutes), but have the disadvantage of adverse reactions (renal failure, coagulopathy and anaphylaxis) and mixing in 0.9% NaCl. Newer 'balanced' gelatins and starches (e.g. 6% Tetraspan) have been introduced in perioperative practice, and have yet to be shown to be superior to 'balanced' crystalloids in critical care.

Further reading

- National Institute for Health and Clinical Excellence. *Nutrition Support in Adults: oral nutrition support, enteral tube feeding and parenteral nutrition.* London: National Institute for Health and Clinical Excellence; 2006.

11

How to assess ICU referrals on the ward

Serena Tolhurst-Cleaver

Taking the referral

The assessment starts from when you receive the referral. This is usually done by telephone, but may be undertaken in person, depending on how close the ICU is to the current location of the patient.

For telephone referrals, this may be your only opportunity to talk to the referring team, as they may have been called away (or not considered it necessary to stay) by the time you reach the ward.

Try to find out the following information and gauge the level of urgency for an ICU review:

- the patient's name (this may sound obvious, but the referring team will often launch into the story before divulging a name!)
- the patient's age and date of birth
- the patient's hospital ID number (you may want to look up blood tests and other investigations before visiting the ward)
- a current set of observations
- current blood test results and arterial blood gas results (if these are unavailable, ask the team to send them)
- whether or not the patient has any significant comorbidities

- the reason for the ICU referral (the most complex part) – you need to consider which organs are failing, and whether or not there is any reversibility in the current clinical picture.

If there will be a delay before you review the patient, tell the referring team when you expect to be able to get there, and under what circumstances they should re-contact you. It may be helpful to give specific parameters. Ask the team to pass a urinary catheter and monitor the hourly urine output if this has not already been done.

If the referral sounds urgent or the patient already has failing organ systems, the ICU will usually have a prepared drug box and transfer bag, which it would be appropriate to take to the patient. Try to familiarise yourself with the contents of this bag before you need to use them! If you are unfamiliar with the set-up of the ward you are going to, it may be easier to take this bag and use its contents, rather than searching endless stock rooms on the ward for the equivalent. However, if you do use anything, make sure that you replace it!

If the referral is mainly about an airway problem (e.g. someone with a reduced conscious level not protecting their airway) or a patient in immediate respiratory distress, intubation may be required, and it is therefore appropriate for the patient to be reviewed by someone with advanced airway skills. If you have not completed your basic training in anaesthesia, make sure that you alert someone with anaesthetic training about the referral. In addition, it may be appropriate to take or prepare anaesthetic drugs and ask the on-call operating department practitioner (ODP) for support.

Arriving on the ward

Reviewing patients on the ward can be stressful, as you may be visiting unfamiliar areas of the hospital for the first time. If you have never been to the ward before, it is useful to phone before you set off and ask them to expect you, as many wards are locked out of hours, and your ID badge may not allow you entry (especially, for example, to obstetric wards). Walking the length of the hospital only to stand outside a locked ward ringing the buzzer to an unmanned nurses' station is extremely frustrating!

When you arrive on the ward, try to find a member of the nursing staff, ideally the nurse who is looking after the patient. If possible, also speak to the referring medical team in person. Locate the patient's notes, including the observation charts, fluid balance chart, drug chart and any post-operative pathway if applicable. This may take some time! Once you have these notes in your possession, if possible keep them with you until you have finished assessing the patient and writing in the notes.

Many people will view your appearance on the ward as an indication that the cavalry has arrived. They may consequently breathe a sigh of relief and make a swift exit. If the referring team are not present on the ward, review the patient and then bleep them and discuss the patient.

Assessing the patient

Be systematic. The easiest way to make sure that you have assessed everything you may be expected to tell your consultant/senior colleague about is to perform the assessment similarly to an ICU daily review, which covers an ABCDE approach.

A: airway

A ward patient will not normally be a trauma victim (although this is not unheard of). Probably the most common threat to the airway on hospital wards is a reduced conscious level. If the patient has a Glasgow Coma Scale (GCS) score of 8 or less, they are certainly not protecting their airway, and their airway is threatened even with a GCS score above this. The safety of the airway should also be considered in patients who are vomiting, or who have epistaxis, haemoptysis or swelling.

B: breathing

The first thing to consider is the respiratory rate. While you are checking this, also consider the patient's general respiratory effort. Are they using accessory muscles to breathe, see-sawing, and do they appear anxious or distressed?

If the respiratory rate is above 30 breaths/minute for a prolonged period, the patient's work of breathing is high, and they will tire if this situation does not improve.

Also consider how much oxygen the patient is on, and whether they have had arterial blood gas analysis performed. If not, these are mandatory when assessing a patient for ICU admission. Is the patient coughing and able to expectorate? If so, look at the sputum and ensure that a sample is sent for culture. Consider whether the patient would benefit from humidified oxygen if the secretions are thick or sticky.

Auscultate the chest and review the recent chest X-rays. If necessary, request a new one.

C: circulation

Assess the heart rate, capillary refill time and blood pressure, but also look back at the observation charts and try to ascertain what is 'normal' for the patient.

The best guide to whether or not the blood pressure is adequate is organ and tissue perfusion. Check the hourly urine output and the arterial blood gas for acidosis and a rising lactate level. Does the patient have IV access? Look at the fluid balance chart.

Listen to the heart sounds, feel the peripheral pulses and look at the mucous membranes. Are the peripheries warm, cool or oedematous? Does the patient feel thirsty?

D: disability

Calculate the GCS score and write the component scores in the notes for anyone reviewing the patient later. If the patient is drowsy or agitated, they will certainly be more difficult to manage on the ward, and they may be unable to take oral medications.

Check the glucose level and also examine the drug chart closely, particularly the 'once only' and 'PRN' prescriptions. Has the patient been given large amounts of opiates, benzodiazepines or other sedative drugs?

E: exposure

As well as completing your examination of the patient, look at any surgical wounds and drain outputs (where applicable). What is the patient's temperature and how has it been measured?

Management of the patient

When you have finished assessing the patient, discuss them with the referring team. Your role is to assess the patient's need for higher-level care, so regardless of whether or not the patient is transferred to the ICU, the further management of the patient must be decided by the referring team. You cannot be expected to become an expert in all the hospital specialties overnight! The next priority is to discuss the patient with your consultant or senior colleague. It is usually easiest to do this while you are still on the ward, as you will have the notes and charts to hand.

If you are concerned about the care that the patient is receiving, try not to display your misgivings in front of the patient or relatives. They may already be extremely anxious, and suggesting that the care they are receiving is sub-standard will only make them more frightened and angry. If they are subsequently admitted to the ICU, this will make them more sceptical about the care provided by the hospital generally, and more difficult to communicate with.

Outright criticism of the referring team or ward staff will only make communication with the team more difficult in future, and undermines their confidence in dealing with sick patients, which may lead to inappropriate referrals in the future. Instead, try to give the ward team some useful practical management advice. For example, a patient with pneumonia may improve dramatically if they are sat bolt upright in bed, given high-concentration humidified oxygen and reviewed by the on-call chest physiotherapist.

If you think that the nursing staff are struggling or unused to dealing with this kind of patient, ask whether one of the ICU nurses can be spared to visit the ward and give the nursing staff some practical tips on managing the patient.

Don't leave the ward without . . .

- Making plans to review the patient (if they are not being admitted to the ICU immediately).
- Giving the nursing staff and referring team clear instructions about when to re-contact you.
- Giving the ward team an interim management plan. Be specific (e.g. hourly observations including urine output, repeat ABG in 1 hour, etc.).
- Being aware of the referring team's management plan for the patient (e.g. whether they need imaging, return to theatre, consultant review, discussion with another specialty, etc.). Make sure that the team implement the plan!

And finally . . .

When reviewing patients it is useful to remember that the majority of suitable patients who are referred for consideration for higher-level care will end up being admitted to an HDU/ICU environment during their hospital stay.

Bearing this in mind, if you review a ward patient and decide not to admit them to the unit, make sure that they are handed over to the next shift and regularly reviewed by either the ICU doctors or the outreach team (if the hospital has one).

12

How to assess a trauma patient

Michael Stewart and Shondipon Laha

Introduction

Trauma is the cause of about 18 000 deaths per year in the UK, representing around 3% of the total death rate. However, trauma is the leading cause of death in the UK among individuals aged 15–30 years, and it remains the leading cause in men aged 30–40 years, so is responsible for more years of life lost than any other disease. In addition, for every person who dies as a result of major trauma, two suffer significant permanent disability.

As major trauma patients are typically young, with a history of being previously well, it is common for critical care teams to be involved in their care.

Phases of trauma care

The traditional definition of trauma deaths was provided by Trunkey in 1983, who described a trimodal distribution:
- minutes after injury, death from massive CNS injury
- hours to days after injury, death from haemorrhage
- days to weeks after injury, death from sepsis and multi-organ failure.

The aim of the Advanced Trauma Life Support (ATLS) approach is to prevent the second category of deaths, with the concept of the 'Golden Hour', which aims for an interval of less than 60 minutes between injury and definitive management of the patient.

Arrival and resuscitation

Initial assessment of the trauma patient should follow the ABCDE approach described on the Advanced Trauma Life Support course:

- **A**irway with cervical spine control
- **B**reathing
- **C**irculation and haemorrhage control
- **D**isability
- **E**xposure and evaluation.

Although this is described sequentially, the response to trauma should involve a team, so many of the steps will be performed simultaneously under the overall direction of the team leader. The aim is to swiftly identify and intervene in any life-threatening injuries.

Airway with cervical spine control

- If there is a possibility of cervical spine injury (this will include any victim of significant blunt trauma), the head should be kept in a neutral position by manual support, sandbags and tape, or with a formal head immobilisation device. A semi-rigid collar is an adjunct to this, but is not sufficient to immobilise the head by itself.
- Open the mouth to look for foreign bodies, loose teeth, blood and vomitus. Look for penetrating wounds of the neck, and any bruising or swelling that would indicate blunt trauma. If significant swelling is observed, consider early intubation before the airway becomes completely occluded.
- Secretions and small amounts of vomit can be cleared by suction. Active vomiting may be best managed by log-rolling on to the side.
- If the patient cannot maintain their own airway, the jaw thrust is the manoeuvre of choice, as it involves minimal neck movement compared with the head tilt/chin lift.
- Consider the use of adjuncts (Guedel or nasopharyngeal airway,

bearing in mind that the latter is relatively contraindicated in patients with suspected basal skull fracture).

- Many trauma patients will require rapid sequence intubation (RSI), either to maintain the airway, to facilitate adequate ventilation, or to enable safe transfer to other areas of the hospital.
- Maintaining the head in a neutral position will typically reduce the view on laryngoscopy by one full Cormack and Lehane grade. If intubation is required, ensure that senior help and difficult airway equipment are available.
- A lateral cervical spine X-ray is a normal part of the trauma series, but is not sufficient to clear the cervical spine, even if normal.

Breathing

- Assess breathing rate, depth and effort.
- Look for penetrating chest wounds. If there is the possibility of open pneumothorax, cover the wound with an Ashermann chest seal or occlusive dressing taped on three sides to act as a flutter valve.
- Palpate the trachea to ensure that it lies in the midline. Deviation is an important but late sign of tension pneumothorax or massive haemothorax.
- Reduced air entry to one side can be a sign of haemothorax or pneumothorax, as can changes in percussion note between sides.
- During the resuscitation phase, all trauma patients should receive high-flow oxygen (15 l/min) via a mask with a reservoir bag. If breathing is inadequate, it should be supported by ventilation from a bag valve mask (BVM) or anaesthetic circuit.
- Suspected tension pneumothorax should be decompressed with a large-bore cannula inserted in the mid-clavicular line, second intercostal space. Pneumothorax and haemothorax will require insertion of a formal chest drain.
- A chest X-ray should be routinely performed as part of the trauma resuscitation.

Circulation

- Assess heart rate, blood pressure, and the presence or absence of peripheral pulses.
- Consider the six bleeding points that can produce life-threatening blood loss:

— abdomen
— retroperitoneum
— pelvis
— thorax
— long bone fracture (predominantly femur)
— external.

- External blood loss can often be controlled with pressure and elevation, but other sources commonly require surgical intervention.
- Establish IV access, taking blood for U&E, FBC, clotting and cross-matching as a minimum.
- Give IV fluids to maintain a systolic blood pressure of around 90 mmHg ('permissive hypotension') until bleeding is controlled. More fluids and higher blood pressure are counter-productive and cause more bleeding by dilution of clotting factors. In the case of an isolated head injury, a higher target blood pressure will usually be more appropriate.
- A 12-lead ECG should be performed. Myocardial contusion can cause rhythm changes or ischaemia.
- An A-P pelvic X-ray is the third and last image in the normal 'trauma series.'

Disability

- Assess the Glasgow Coma Scale (GCS) score, pupil response to light, and any focal neurological deficit (check whether the patient can move all four limbs).
- Capillary blood glucose levels should be checked.
- A GCS score of ≤ 8 is an indicator that the airway will need to be protected by intubation.
- Any reduction in GCS score or focal neurological deficit in trauma is an indication for CT imaging of the head and cervical spine.

Expose and evaluate

- Complete exposure and assessment for further significant injuries should complete the primary survey.
- The patient should be log-rolled to examine the back, including PR examination for blood (which suggests bowel injury), high-riding prostate (which indicates pelvic fracture) and anal tone (if reduced or absent, this indicates spinal trauma).

- Ensure that the patient is re-covered and kept warm as soon as possible.
- A full secondary survey is required at some point for all significant trauma patients, but should not delay life-saving interventions.

In addition to the physical assessment, a brief focused history should be taken. The AMPLE mnemonic provides a useful way to approach this:

- **A**llergies
- **M**edications currently taken
- **P**ast medical history
- **L**ast food and drink
- **E**vents (i.e. mechanism of injury).

Transfer

A decision needs to be made swiftly as to where the patient should be transferred. The critical care doctor will often be involved in monitoring the patient and ensuring a safe transfer.

- If the patient is haemodynamically unstable, they require urgent transfer to a setting that permits control of bleeding. If intra-abdominal bleeding is known or suspected, this setting will be an operating theatre for laparotomy. In some injuries (e.g. bleeding associated with pelvic fractures), angiography and embolisation may be more appropriate.
- If the patient is haemodynamically stable, they will often require further imaging, typically CT, to determine the extent of injuries and to guide further management.
- If no operative intervention is needed, the patient will require transfer to the ICU or ward, depending on the injuries found and the overall status.

Ongoing critical care

The initial resuscitation of the trauma patient focuses on anatomy – identifying and correcting life-threatening bleeding. Once this has been addressed, physiology takes precedence over more minor injuries. To a greater or lesser extent, all victims of serious trauma are hypothermic, acidotic and coagulopathic. This triad is lethal unless appropriately addressed, and it is here that good-quality critical care treatment saves lives in trauma patients.

Hypothermia

- Trauma often involves a period of exposure to the environment and some resultant hypothermia.
- Infusion of fluids below body temperature will exacerbate this.
- Shock and hypoperfusion of tissues that normally generate heat prevent the body from restoring the normal core temperature.
- Prevention of heat loss at all stages, with blankets and warm resuscitation and operating areas, is the first step.
- Rewarming with warm air blankets and, if hypothermia is severe, invasive methods such as peritoneal, pleural and bladder lavage with warmed fluids may be required.

Acidosis

- Reduced tissue perfusion as a result of blood loss leads to anaerobic metabolism.
- Correction of acidosis is best achieved by careful attention to optimisation of tissue perfusion.
- This will require a combination of fluid infusion, transfusion, and often inotropes and vasopressors.

Coagulopathy

- Tissue injury will cause activation of the coagulation cascade and a degree of disseminated intravascular coagulation (DIC).
- Blood loss and infusion of fluids will cause loss and dilution of clotting factors, respectively.
- Even after major bleeds have been addressed, coagulopathy will lead to ongoing uncontrolled ooze.
- In massive transfusion (> 10 units of red cells in 24 hours expected), clotting factors will be depleted, and transfusion of 1 unit of FFP for each unit of red cells is advised, with one pooled unit of platelets for every 4 units of red cells.
- Cryoprecipitate and specific factor concentrates may also be required, and close liaison with the haematology department is advisable.

There is a mounting body of evidence that significant injuries are regularly missed in the primary and secondary surveys of trauma patients. These can be life-threatening, limb-threatening and function-threatening. It is easy to miss a fractured finger in the rush to stabilise a patient with a hepatic laceration, but if the patient otherwise makes a full recovery, the minor injury that, for example, prevents them from resuming their career as a concert pianist will have a disproportionate effect on their livelihood, and carries a risk of future legal action.

The 'tertiary survey' has been described as a further systematic examination of the trauma patient in the critical care unit, aimed at identifying all injuries. It consists of the following:

- consideration of the mechanism of injury and the resultant likely injury patterns
- review of all known injuries and re-evaluation of the management plan for these, to confirm that it is still appropriate
- a full secondary survey, including rolling the patient to inspect the back, assessment of limbs (including the digits), and assessment of function if the patient is conscious
- further imaging guided by the examination to investigate the potential injuries
- establishment of a management plan for all injuries, in conjunction with other specialties as required.

Further reading

- American College of Surgeons. *Advanced Trauma Life Support for Doctors*. 8th edn. Chicago, IL: American College of Surgeons; 2008.
- National Confidential Enquiry into Patient Outcome and Death. *Trauma: who cares?* London: National Confidential Enquiry into Patient Outcome and Death; 2007.

13

The head-injured patient

Peter Duncan

Patients with head injuries are often young and in good health. Failure to achieve the best possible outcome for a brain injury has catastrophic consequences for the patient, their family and society. Although specific management of the injured brain is very important, it is attention to the details of maintaining the best supportive care which can make a huge difference to the outcome. The emphasis in this chapter will be on the initial assessment and treatment of head injury, without considering the longer-term neurosurgical and intensive care management of brain injury.

As with all assessments of sick patients, a structured approach is advocated for head-injured patients.

A: airway

- Remember that a neck injury may be present.
- Give oxygen at a rate of 15 litres/minute via a face mask with a reservoir bag.
- Make sure that the airway is clear and not obstructed.
- An obstructed airway will cause both hypoxia and a raised blood carbon dioxide level.

- A low oxygen level will further damage injured brain cells.
- A raised carbon dioxide level will increase cerebral blood flow, leading to an increased intracranial pressure (ICP).
- If the airway cannot be maintained by airway manoeuvres or by inserting an oral airway, intubate the patient.

B: breathing

- Are the rate and depth of respiration adequate?
- Bag-and-mask ventilate the patient if breathing is inadequate, and get anaesthetic help.
- Check whether there are other associated injuries (e.g. pneumothorax, lung contusions).
- Insert a chest drain if necessary to drain a pneumothorax or haemothorax.
- A raised carbon dioxide level will increase cerebral blood flow, leading to an increased ICP.
- A low oxygen level will further damage injured brain cells.
- Check whether the patient is hyperventilating.
- Consider intubation and controlled ventilation.

C: circulation

- Check the pulse and blood pressure.
- Give fluid to restore these parameters to normal.
- Does the patient respond to fluid resuscitation?
- Are the patient's pulse and blood pressure maintained without further fluid?
- Is the patient bleeding?
- Control bleeding, and obtain a surgical review.
- If there is major haemorrhage, remember to cross-match the patient.

D: disability

- Determine the Glasgow Coma Scale (GCS) score.
- Alternatively, determine the Alert, Voice, Pain, Unresponsive (AVPU) score.
- If the GCS score is ≤ 8, or the AVPU score is P, the patient requires intubation and ventilation.
- Check the size and reaction of the pupils.

- If the patient has a low GCS score and dilated pupil(s), give 200 ml of 20% mannitol.
- Check whether there are any signs or a history of fitting.
- Treat pain with morphine if required.
- It is acceptable for head-injured patients to be mildly hypothermic, so do not actively rewarm the patient.

E: exposure

- Check for other injuries, especially sources of possible bleeding.
- Check whether there is blood or cerebrospinal fluid (CSF) coming from the nose or ears, which suggests a base of skull fracture.

TABLE 13.1 Glasgow Coma Scale

BEST MOTOR RESPONSE	SCORE
Obeys commands	6
Localises to pain	5
Withdraws from pain	4
Abnormal flexion	3
Decorticate posturing	2
No response	1
BEST VERBAL RESPONSE	
Orientated	5
Confused	4
Inappropriate speech	3
Incomprehensible sounds	2
None	1
BEST EYE OPENING	
Spontaneous	4
To speech	3

Further investigation

- A CT scan of the head and neck is required. Although this is necessary, the patient must be safely prepared and stabilised before being transferred to the scanner.
- Do not be pressurised into taking the patient before you are ready.

- Secure the airway. If you have not been trained to perform a rapid sequence induction (RSI), get help.
- Ensure that the endotracheal tube is correctly placed by auscultating the chest and attaching a capnograph to measure end tidal carbon dioxide (CO_2).
- Check that the transfer ventilator is charged, has sufficient oxygen and is attached and functioning at the appropriate settings to maintain mild hypocarbia.
- Sedate the patient with an opiate (e.g. morphine) and a hypnotic (e.g. propofol), and paralyse with a non-depolarising muscle relaxant (e.g. atracurium).

Ongoing care

- Assuming that there is no reason for the patient to undergo neurosurgical intervention, move them to the critical care unit.
- Nurse the patient with a 30° head-up tilt.
- Keep them sedated with an opioid analgesic and a sedative. Muscle relaxants are not mandatory.
- Insert arterial and central venous lines if these are not already in place.
- Avoid hypoxia, but also avoid high levels of positive end-expiratory pressure (PEEP), as these may inhibit venous return and raise ICP.
- Maintain mild hypocarbia ($PaCO_2$ 4.0–4.5 kPa).
- Maintain blood pressure to ensure an adequate cerebral perfusion pressure (CPP).
- Keep the patient well hydrated.
- Use noradrenaline if the CPP is still low despite adequate fluid resuscitation.
- Catheterise the patient if this has not already been done.
- Insert a nasogastric tube if there are no signs of basal skull fracture, or an orogastric tube if these signs are present (e.g. bleeding from the ears, CSF coming from the ears or nose).
- Ensure that the ties securing the endotracheal tube are not too tight, as they will impede venous drainage from the head, resulting in an increase in ICP.
- Avoid pyrexia.
- Do not actively warm the patient if they are mildly hypothermic.
- Treat raised intracranial pressure with 200 ml of 20% mannitol in an emergency to buy time for neurosurgical intervention.

14

Initial management of the patient with burns

Thomas Owen

Key points

- Adopt an 'ATLS' approach.
- A good history of the accident is essential.
- Anticipate and treat airway problems early.
- Do not miss associated injuries.

History

- Time.
- Mechanism:
  — risk of associated injuries
  — enclosed space – assume carbon monoxide (CO) poisoning
  — electrical burns – a small burn can cause significant internal injury
  — exposure to chemicals.

Primary survey

A: airway

- Cervical spine immobilisation.
- Risk of airway injury and compromise if any of the following are present:
  — stridor/hoarse voice
  — soot in nares, mouth and/or sputum
  — facial burns
  — singed facial and/or nasal hair.
- Low threshold for intubation – oedema can progress rapidly, so summon experienced anaesthetic help, as intubation can be difficult.
- **Always** use uncut endotracheal tube.

B: breathing (and burning)

- **Remove all burnt clothing.** This stops the burning process. Care is needed if there is a history of chemical exposure.
- **Give 100% O_2.** Assume that carbon monoxide (CO) poisoning has occurred if there is a history of being in an enclosed space. Check the CO levels on arterial blood gas analysis. Oxygen reduces the half-life of CO.
- **Normal pulse oximetry does not exclude CO poisoning.**
- **Inhalational injury.** This progresses over a period of hours. The risk factors are the same as for airway injury.

C: circulation

- Establish good IV access, if necessary through burnt skin.
- Estimate the patient's fluid requirements using the Parkland formula (**4 ml of Hartmann's solution/kg body weight/% body surface area burnt over 24 hours – give half in the first 8 hours**).
- Calculate from time of the burn, **not** from the time of admission.
- Adjust fluids according to clinical response. Catheterise and aim for a urine output of 0.5–1.0 ml/kg/hour.

D: disability

- Determine the GCS score.
- If it is low, consider the following:
  — associated head injury
  — CO poisoning
  — other inhaled toxins.

- Analgesia – titrate small IV morphine boluses to effect.

E: exposure
- **Keep the patient warm.** Hypothermia must be avoided, so use warming blankets, warmed IV fluids, etc.
- **Cover burns with cling film.** If you are unsure, discuss with burns centre.
- **Ascertain the patient's tetanus status.**

Assess depth of burns
- **Simple erythema** – 'sunburn.'
- **Superficial partial thickness** – blisters, very painful.
- **Deep partial thickness** – whiter, less painful.
- **Full thickness** – leathery, painless.

Assess extent of burns
'Rule of nines'
- Exclude simple erythema.
- Needs to be adjusted for children.
- **Head: 9%.**
- **Arm: 9%.**
- **Leg: 18%.**
- **Torso: front, 18%; back, 18%.**
- **Perineum: 1%.**

Circumferential burns
- **Torso** – respiratory compromise.
- **Limbs** – compartment syndrome.
- These burns require escharotomy.

Indications for referral to burns centre
- Partial-thickness burns > 10% of total body surface area (> 5% in children).
- Any full-thickness burn.

- Burns to the face, hands, feet, perineum or major joints.
- Inhalational injury.
- Electrical and chemical burns.

15

Maintaining an airway

Nitin Arora

Maintaining an airway is a life-saving procedure with which all doctors should be familiar. Critically ill patients, especially those who require resuscitation, often have an obstructed airway. This is usually caused by loss of consciousness.

Causes of airway obstruction

Obstruction of the upper airways may be partial or complete. In the unconscious patient, this is generally due to loss of pharyngeal muscle tone. It may also be caused by vomit, blood from trauma, or by a foreign body.

Laryngeal obstruction may be caused by trauma, inflammation or burns.

Recognising an obstructed airway

- This is best managed by the look, listen and feel approach.
- **Look** for chest and abdomen movements.
- **Listen** and **feel** for air coming out of the mouth and nose, and for any added sounds.

- Added sounds may be due to partial airway obstruction, and may include stridor, gurgling or snoring.

Basic airway opening manoeuvres

After recognising airway obstruction, the next step is to relieve it. The main manoeuvres used are as follows:
- head tilt
- chin lift
- jaw thrust.

Head tilt and chin lift

Place one hand on the patient's forehead, and use the other hand to gently lift the chin. This is generally successful, but must not be attempted if there is cervical spine instability, in which case the jaw thrust technique should be tried.

Jaw thrust

Locate the angle of the mandible and then, with the fingers under the angle, apply upward pressure while opening the mouth with the thumbs.

Reassess the airway by looking, listening and feeling after each manoeuvre, to assess success.

If a clear airway is not achieved, look for other causes of obstruction (e.g. foreign bodies, vomit, etc.).

Airway adjuncts

If the above basic techniques have not been successful, oropharyngeal or nasopharyngeal airways may be tried.

The oropharyngeal (Guedel) airway is a curved plastic tube with a flange at the end. It must be sized appropriately before insertion. Its length should be the distance between the patient's incisors and the angle of the jaw.

For insertion of this device, open the mouth and insert the airway 'upside down' until it reaches the soft palate. Rotate it through 180° and then advance it again until it is in the pharynx. The flattened portion should sit between the patient's teeth.

After insertion, reassess the airway as described above.

The nasopharyngeal airway is a soft plastic tube with a bevel at one end and a flange at the other. It is better tolerated than the Guedel airway by patients who are not deeply unconscious. Sizes 6–7 are suitable for most adults. Lubricate the airway and then insert the airway gently into the nose with a twisting motion. Some flanges may require the insertion of a safety pin to avoid the airway being lost into the nose. *If so, be carful not to stab the patient with the safety pin.*

This airway must not be used in a suspected base of skull fracture.

Once the airway is in place, reassess it as described earlier.

Chin lift, head tilt and jaw thrust may still be needed in conjunction with these airways.

Ventilation

If the patient is not breathing despite an open airway, artificial ventilation must be started. Mouth-to-mouth and pocket-mask ventilation are options, but in a hospital setting you would generally have access to a self-inflating bag and mask. We recommend a two-person technique where one person holds the mask on the patient's face with jaw thrust while the assistant squeezes the bag. This enables a better seal and more effective ventilation.

Using a bag and mask requires skill and practice, but can be extremely useful for resuscitation.

Advanced airways

Laryngeal mask airways (LMA) and endotracheal tubes provide a better airway with more effective ventilation, but discussion of their insertion and use is beyond the scope of this book.

16

What to do if the endotracheal tube or tracheostomy falls out

Kenneth McGrattan and Brendan McGrath

These are potentially stressful situations where quick action is required to prevent anoxic brain damage or cardiac arrest.

The diagnosis is not always obvious. Partially dislodged endotracheal tubes (ETT) or tracheostomies are more difficult to manage than complete tube displacement.

Always consider the diagnosis in a distressed, tachypnoeic patient with an endotracheal tube or tracheostomy *in situ*.

Endotracheal tube displacement
Key points
- Don't panic.
- Give 100% oxygen.
- Call for anaesthetic/intensive care help early.
- Reassure the patient.

Intubated patients may be breathing spontaneously via the ETT or they may be completely ventilator dependent and not able to initiate their own

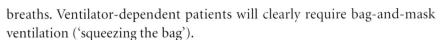

breaths. Ventilator-dependent patients will clearly require bag-and-mask ventilation ('squeezing the bag').

The key steps involved in the initial management of the intubated patient with breathing difficulties are described below.

Endotracheal tube removed from the mouth

1 Call anaesthetist for help.
2 Open the airway using head tilt (if there is no history of trauma), chin lift and jaw thrust.
   - Is breathing (if present) noisy? If so, suction the airway.
   - An oropharyngeal, nasopharyngeal or laryngeal mask airway (LMA) may be required to open the airway. Only insert these if you have been trained in their use.
3 Apply a tight-fitting face mask over the patient's mouth and nose and attach a Water's circuit (see below).
   - If an LMA has been inserted, attach the Water's circuit to this.
   - If the patient is not breathing (i.e. the bag is not moving), attempt to ventilate by squeezing the bag.
   - Check oxygen saturations.
   - Does the bag move with the patient's respiration or does the chest move as you squeeze the bag? Is a capnograph trace (see below) present?
   - If not, it is not possible to maintain an airway.
4 Feel for a pulse. If this is not present, start CPR according to UK Resuscitation Council guidelines. If a pulse is present, check the blood pressure.
5 If the airway is maintained, oxygenation is adequate and the patient is cardiovascularly stable, a decision will be made with the senior anaesthetist/intensivist as to whether the ETT needs to be replaced.
6 If it is impossible to maintain an airway or keep the patient oxygenated, the ETT will need to be replaced following rapid sequence induction by an anaesthetist.
7 Very rarely it is impossible to maintain an airway or replace the ETT (i.e. 'can't intubate, can't ventilate').
   - The Difficult Airway Society has developed guidelines for management of this scenario.
   - An experienced anaesthetist must be present to deal with this situation.

Endotracheal tube remains in the mouth

1 Call anaesthetist for help.
2 Look, listen and feel for breathing at the end of the ETT.
3 If this is not present, attach a Water's circuit and give high-flow oxygen.
   - Check oxygen saturations.
   - Does the bag move with the patient's respiration, or does the chest move as you squeeze the bag? Is a capnograph trace present?
4 If not, remove the ETT from the airway. Now use the guideline for ETT removed from the mouth.
5 If the chest moves with attempted ventilation with a bag, and a consistent capnograph trace is present, the ETT is in the trachea.
   - Continue bag ventilation with high-flow oxygen, monitor oxygen saturations and look for other causes of respiratory distress (pneumothorax, sputum plug, pulmonary oedema, 'fighting the ventilator').
6 Check the pulse and blood pressure.

Mapleson C circuit

This is a bag-and-valve device (*see* Figure 16.1) that can be connected to a mask or airway device. Spontaneous breathing can be monitored by bag movement, and positive pressure ventilation can be given by manually squeezing the bag.

Capnography

This is the measurement of carbon dioxide levels in expired gases. A typical capnograph trace from a breathing circuit is shown in Figure 16.2. A consistent trace can only come from the lungs.

Tracheostomy tube emergencies

Tracheostomies are performed by ENT and maxillofacial surgeons in theatre, and by intensivists on critical care units. They are becoming more common on open wards.

Tracheostomy patients with breathing difficulties may have:
- a problem with their airway: tracheostomy (blocked, complete or partial removal)
- other 'breathing problems': (pneumothorax, exacerbation of COPD, pulmonary oedema).

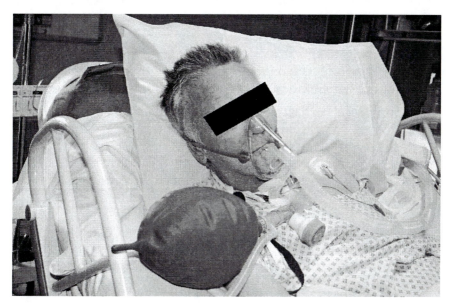

FIGURE 16.1

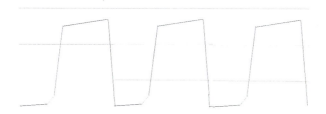

FIGURE 16.2

Key points

- Don't panic.
- Maintain an airway and keep the patient oxygenated.
- Apply 100% oxygen to both face **and** tracheostomy stoma.
- Call for senior anaesthetic/intensive care and ENT/maxillofacial assistance early on.
- Essential airway and tracheostomy equipment must be at the bedside. Call for advanced equipment (e.g. fibre-optic scopes) early on, and be aware of where they are kept.

- Reassure the patient.
- Bag-and-mask ventilation via the mouth is not usually possible with a cuffed tracheostomy tube *in situ* unless the tracheostomy is displaced.
- Bag-and-mask ventilation via the mouth is not possible if the patient has had a laryngectomy, as there is no communication between the upper airways and the trachea.

Tracheostomy basics

A tracheotomy is an artificial opening which has been surgically (or percutaneously) formed in the anterior trachea, which allows a stoma to be created from the skin of the anterior neck to the trachea – the tracheostomy. Tubes may be inserted through this stoma to allow:

- connection to an anaesthetic breathing circuit (e.g. Water's circuit)
- a cuff to be inflated in order to:
  — 'seal off' the pharynx and upper airway (reducing the risk of aspiration)
  — allow positive pressure to be administered
- suctioning and 'airway toilet' to be performed without traumatising the soft tissues.

A tracheostomy stoma does not always have a tracheostomy tube inserted into it. The tubes are described in terms of the following characteristics:

- their internal diameter
- their length (some are adjustable to allow their use in patients with larger necks)
- the presence of a cuff
- the presence of an inner removable cannula which reduces the risk of the tube becoming blocked with secretions
- the presence of a 'fenestration' or hole in the tube to allow air to move upwards through the larynx, which can allow the patient to talk.

Surgical and percutaneous tracheostomies
Surgical tracheostomies

- The anterior portions of two tracheal rings are removed.
- Usually there is a single-lumen adjustable flange (see below).
- The stoma may be stitched open and the 'stay sutures' brought up to the skin surface to aid tube re-insertion.

- Easier to re-insert than percutaneous tracheostomies, especially after 3 days post-procedure.

Percutaneous tracheostomies
- Insertion involves a dilatational Seldinger wire technique.
- There may be a single or double lumen.
- More difficult to re-insert before 7–10 days post-procedure.

Single or double lumen
Double-lumen tubes
- These have inner and outer cannulae (*see* Figure 16.3).
- The inner cannula can be easily removed for cleaning, or if the tube becomes obstructed.

Single-lumen tubes
- There is no inner cannula, so the tube is at increased risk of blockage.
- Some are fixed to the neck by a flange, which can be adjustable for larger necks (*see* Figure 16.4).

Cuffed or uncuffed
- A cuff is an air-filled sac that lies around the tip of the tube, separating the lungs from the upper airway.
- The cuff is inflated via the pilot tube.
- It is not possible to ventilate the lungs effectively through an uncuffed tracheostomy or a cuffed tracheostomy with a deflated cuff.

Fenestrated or unfenestrated inner tube
- Fenestrated inner tubes have small holes on their superior aspect that allow air to pass through and therefore allow the patient to speak.
- It is not possible to effectively ventilate the lungs through a fenestrated tube.

Laryngectomy patients
During a laryngectomy the larynx is removed and the trachea is stitched to the anterior neck. These patients have no communication between the oral/nasal cavities and the trachea/lungs, so they cannot be oxygenated or

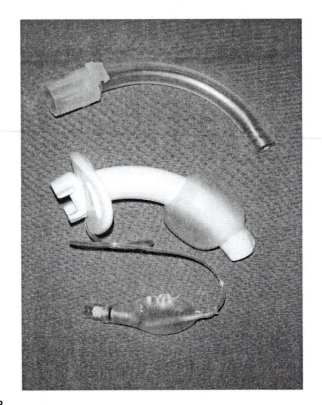

FIGURE 16.3

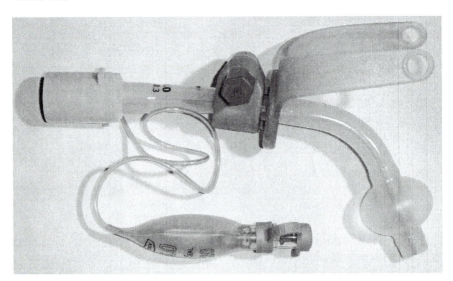

FIGURE 16.4

ventilated via the nose or mouth. In these patients, oxygen must be applied to the tracheal stoma, and any attempts at ventilation must occur via this stoma.

Mini-tracheostomy

This is usually inserted through the cricothyroid membrane to allow suctioning of secretions. It can be used to 'downsize' a tracheostomy stoma when a tracheostomy tube is removed, either to keep a tract open (if the tracheostomy might need to be re-inserted) or to provide help with secretion management when ventilation is no longer required. The lack of a cuff and the narrow lumen preclude its use for mechanical ventilation, although oxygen can be administered if necessary.

Managing tracheostomy emergencies

Tracheostomy patients may present with worrying or red flag signs. These may herald a sudden deterioration and require urgent review by an experienced doctor. Red flags include the following:

- increasing ventilator support or increasing oxygen requirements
- respiratory distress
- the patient suddenly being able to talk, or 'bubbling' of secretions in the mouth (indicating that gas is escaping proximally and the cuff is no longer 'sealing' the trachea)
- frequent requirement for (excessive) inflation of the cuff to prevent air leak
- pain at the tracheostomy site
- surgical (subcutaneous) emphysema (gas in the soft tissues)
- the patient complaining that they cannot breathe or that they have difficulties in breathing
- a suction catheter not passing easily into the trachea
- a changing, inadequate or absent capnograph trace
- suspicion of aspiration (feed aspirated on tracheal toilet, which suggests that the cuff is not functioning adequately).

Algorithms

Two algorithms for the management of the tracheostomy patient with breathing difficulties are presented on pages 86 and 87.

- It is important to distinguish patients with a patent upper airway from those without one (laryngectomy patients).
- Oxygen should be applied to both the face and stoma. This will require two oxygen sources.
- Anaesthetics/critical care and ENT/maxillofacial surgery should be called urgently, and a bronchoscope should be requested urgently.
- A key step is to decide whether the patient's respiratory distress is due to blockage, displacement or some other cause (e.g. pneumothorax).
- Inflating the tracheostomy tube cuff (if present) provides the best method of detecting spontaneous breathing and assessing whether the tracheostomy tube is patent. Look, listen and feel for breath at the tube end, look for movement of a Water's circuit when attached to the tracheostomy, look for a capnograph trace, and look at the patient's chest.
- If it is not possible to pass a suction catheter, the cuff should be deflated, as this may allow a spontaneously breathing patient to breathe around a blocked or displaced tube.
- If an inner tube is present, it should be removed, unblocked and replaced.
- Reassess breathing at the mouth/nose and the tracheostomy.
- If the patient is not breathing and the tracheostomy is not patent (a suction catheter will not pass), vigorous attempts at ventilation may make the situation worse by causing surgical emphysema.
- If this does not result in improvement, the tracheostomy should be removed (unless an airway expert is present and safe adequate oxygenation is occurring via the facial route, in which case the tracheostomy may be manipulated).
- The patient may now require orotracheal intubation, re-intubation of the stoma, or the use of other airway adjuncts (e.g. laryngeal mask airway). The decision as to which is the most appropriate will depend upon the following:
  — the anticipated difficulty of orotracheal intubation
  — whether a track is well formed (at least 72 hours for a surgical tracheostomy and 7–10 days for a percutaneous one)
  — the doctor's skills
  — the level of clinical urgency.
- The goal is a stable, oxygenated patient. If you do not have the skills to safely insert a tracheostomy tube or an endotracheal tube, and the patient is stable, wait for an expert.

Expert tips

- An LMA or paediatric face mask applied to the stoma can be an effective seal and allow ventilation without a tracheostomy tube.
- Sedating a spontaneously breathing, stable patient can be extremely dangerous if they have a difficult upper airway and tracheostomy. This should only be done if the right skills, equipment and personnel are available, and it may require a trip to theatre in order to be done safely.
- An Aintree catheter loaded on to a fibre-optic bronchoscope is much better than trying to poke a bougie or similar instrument into a precarious stoma.

Further reading

- Resuscitation Council (UK). *Adult Basic Life Support Guidelines 2005.* www.resus.org.uk/pages/bls.pdf (accessed 22 February 2010).
- Resuscitation Council (UK). *Adult Advanced Life Support Guidelines 2005.* www.resus.org.uk/pages/als.pdf (accessed 22 February 2010).
- *Difficult Airway Society Failed Ventilation Guidelines.* www.das.uk.com/guidelines/cvci.html (accessed 14 February 2010).
- North West Regional Tracheostomy Group website: www.tracheostomy.org.uk (accessed 14 February 2010).
- Intensive Care Society (2008) *Standards for the Care of Adult Patients with a Temporary Tracheostomy.* www.ics.ac.uk/icmprof/downloads/ICS Tracheostomy standards.pdf (accessed 14 February 2010).

Management of the tracheostomy patient with breathing difficulties: patent upper airway

100% O_2 applied to **both** the face and the tracheostomy stoma
Call for help – Anaesthetics/ITU *and* ENT/Max Fax

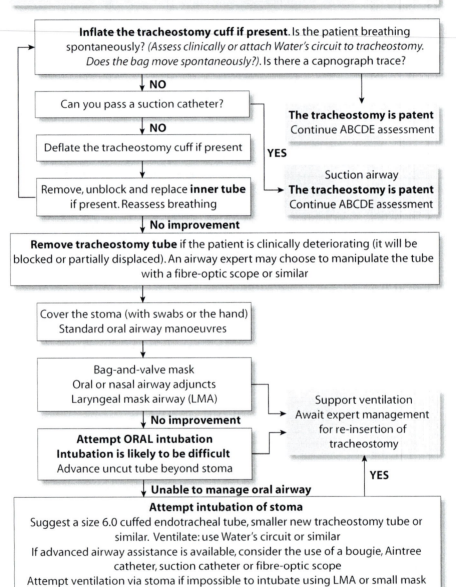

Inflate the tracheostomy cuff if present. Is the patient breathing spontaneously? *(Assess clinically or attach Water's circuit to tracheostomy. Does the bag move spontaneously?).* Is there a capnograph trace?

↓ **NO**

Can you pass a suction catheter?

↓ **NO**

Deflate the tracheostomy cuff if present

Remove, unblock and replace **inner tube** if present. Reassess breathing

The tracheostomy is patent
Continue ABCDE assessment

YES

Suction airway
The tracheostomy is patent
Continue ABCDE assessment

↓ **No improvement**

Remove tracheostomy tube if the patient is clinically deteriorating (it will be blocked or partially displaced). An airway expert may choose to manipulate the tube with a fibre-optic scope or similar

Cover the stoma (with swabs or the hand)
Standard oral airway manoeuvres

Bag-and-valve mask
Oral or nasal airway adjuncts
Laryngeal mask airway (LMA)

Support ventilation
Await expert management
for re-insertion of
tracheostomy

↓ **No improvement**

Attempt ORAL intubation
Intubation is likely to be difficult
Advance uncut tube beyond stoma

YES

↓ **Unable to manage oral airway**

Attempt intubation of stoma
Suggest a size 6.0 cuffed endotracheal tube, smaller new tracheostomy tube or similar. Ventilate: use Water's circuit or similar
If advanced airway assistance is available, consider the use of a bougie, Aintree catheter, suction catheter or fibre-optic scope
Attempt ventilation via stoma if impossible to intubate using LMA or small mask applied to skin

Management of the tracheostomy patient with breathing difficulties: laryngectomy

100% O_2 applied to **both** the face and the tracheostomy stoma*
Call for help – Anaesthetics/ITU *and* ENT/Max Fax

Inflate the tracheostomy cuff if present. If there is no tracheostomy tube, proceed to suction. Is the patient breathing spontaneously? *(Assess clinically or attach Water's circuit to tracheostomy. Does the bag move spontaneously?)*
Is there a capnograph trace?

NO → → **YES**

Can you pass a suction catheter?

NO

Deflate the tracheostomy cuff if present

YES

Remove, unblock and replace inner tube if present. **Reassess breathing**

The tracheostomy is patent
Continue ABCDE assessment

Suction airway
The tracheostomy is patent
Continue ABCDE assessment

No improvement

Remove tracheostomy tube if the patient is clinically deteriorating (it will be blocked or partially displaced). An airway expert may choose to manipulate the tube with a fibre-optic scope or similar

Apply a small face mask to the stoma (try a paediatric mask or LMA)
Is the patient breathing spontaneously?
Can you ventilate adequately?

YES →

Support ventilation
Await expert management for re-insertion of tracheostomy

YES

No improvement

Attempt intubation of stoma
Suggest a size 6.0 cuffed endotracheal tube, smaller new tracheostomy tube or similar
Ventilate: use Water's circuit or similar
If advanced airway assistance is available, consider the use of a bougie, Aintree catheter, suction catheter or fibre-optic scope
Attempt ventilation via stoma if impossible to intubate stoma using LMA or small mask applied to skin

---

Laryngectomy patients have an end stoma and no communication between the mouth and the trachea.
***Applying oxygen to the face and neck is a default emergency action for all patients with a tracheostomy.**

17

'Fighting the ventilator'

James Wilson

'Fighting' is the term used to describe a number of causes of poor ventilation in a previously stable mechanically ventilated patient. This can happen when a patient becomes agitated, sedation levels fall or they try to breathe out of sync with the ventilator, also known as dyssynchrony. Each of these problems will cause a rise in airways pressure and ultimately a fall in minute volume, leading to hypoxia and hypercarbia.

> 'Your patient in Bed 4 is "fighting" the ventilator. Could you please review him?'

The structured approach to this request can be divided into two phases, namely initial assessment and resuscitation, followed by identification of the problem.

Initial assessment

An immediate decision about the severity of the problem should be made. Is oxygenation of the patient compromised? Is ventilation so poor that carbon dioxide levels are too high? Hypoxia and hypercarbia are emergency situations and should be dealt with in a structured 'ABC' manner as described below. Several actions will occur simultaneously, and problems should be treated in the order in which they are identified.

- Call for help.
- Administer 100% oxygen.
- A: check the position of the ET tube, and ensure that there are no kinks or blockages.
- B: disconnect the ventilator and, using a self-inflating bag or Water's circuit, ventilate by hand with 100% oxygen. Is ventilation adequate? Can you hear breath sounds bilaterally? Is chest expansion adequate?
- C: check whether blood pressure and heart rate are haemodynamically stable.

Identification of the problem

If the patient is stable and there is no emergency treatment required, or once the patient has been successfully resuscitated, troubleshooting to identify the cause of 'fighting' can commence. This can be divided into three broad areas, namely circuit/ventilator, intrathoracic and patient problems.

Circuit/ventilator problems

Starting with the patient, work back along the circuit towards the ventilator.

- **ET tube.** Is it blocked (due to kinks or secretions)? Has it travelled into the right main bronchus? Reintubate if necessary.
- **Circuit.** Is the circuit kinked? Are there any pools of fluid causing increased resistance? Check for disconnections. If the circuit has any problems, switch to manual ventilation with a self-inflating bag/Water's circuit.
- **Ventilator.** Is the ventilator on the correct setting? Could the setting be reduced as part of weaning? Are the alarm limits appropriate?

Intrathoracic problems

Examine the chest: auscultate, palpate and percuss.

- Wheeze on auscultation indicates bronchospasm. Identify the cause and treat with bronchodilators.

- Crepitations indicate pulmonary oedema. Assess fluid balance, consider diuretics, and treat the cause.
- Consolidation due to infection; treat pneumonia empirically.
- Reduced air entry/unequal chest movements may be due to:
  — haemothorax or pneumothorax (increased risk with high airway pressures): chest drain, chest X-ray
  — pleural effusion: chest X-ray, may require draining
  — lobar collapse: chest X-ray, investigatation of cause, check whether the tube is in the right main bronchus.

Patient problems

- First ask yourself whether the patient requires the current level of ventilator support. Patients should have a weaning plan, and it may be that your patient can be weaned to the next level of support.
- If they still require this level of ventilation, can it be delivered in a more comfortable manner? Could they be switched to a synchronised setting, as these are usually better tolerated?
- Is the patient appropriately sedated? Simply increasing the sedation level may help the patient to tolerate the ventilator. The sedation may need to be changed, depending on your department's protocols.
- Finally, rule out other causes of discomfort/agitation. Any degree of pain can cause a patient to 'fight' the ventilator. They may have a full bladder or bowel that is causing considerable discomfort, or invasive lines or monitoring, or even the ET tube position may be causing irritation.

Conclusion

Maintaining oxygenation followed by adequate ventilation is your primary goal. Once the patient is stable, you can troubleshoot the problem. Taking a structured approach allows you to identify and treat potential causes as you find them. If the patient still fights the ventilator and their clinical condition requires high levels of ventilator support, adequate sedation and use of muscle relaxants may be your only option.

18

Pneumothorax

Amanda Shaw

Definition

Pneumothorax is a collection of air in the space *around* the lungs – that is, between the lungs and the chest wall (i.e. between the visceral and parietal pleura). This is not the right place for air to be!

What causes pneumothorax?

A tiny tear in an outer part of the lung allows air to escape and become trapped between the lung and the chest wall.

1 Spontaneous pneumothorax:
   - primary:
     — no apparent cause
     — occurs mainly in healthy young people
     — occurs in 18–28 in 100 000 young men, and < 6 in 100 000 young women
     — unusual in individuals over 40 years of age
   - secondary:
     — underlying lung problem

— occurs in patients with asthma, COPD, pneumonia, TB, sarcoidosis, cystic fibrosis, lung cancer and pulmonary fibrosis.

2 Other:
- external trauma
- internal trauma, e.g. high pressures generated by breathing machine (ventilator) if patient is mechanically ventilated
- some surgical operations.

Detection of pneumothorax

The patient may:
- complain of sudden sharp chest pain followed by pains when they breathe in (pleuritic chest pain)
- appear short of breath.

Observation of patient

- Hypoxia (low oxygen saturations) may suddenly develop.
- The patient may appear cyanosed (blue).
- The patient may start to breathe more rapidly or appear to find it difficult to breathe (respiratory distress).
- The blood pressure may fall and the heart rate may rise.
- You may be able to see distended neck veins on the patient.
- There may be an increase in the central venous pressure (CVP)
- The trachea may be pushed away from the side of the pneumothorax.
- If the patient is being ventilated (on a breathing machine), their breathing pattern may appear to 'fight' the ventilator.
- Ventilator pressures may suddenly and inexplicably rise.

Examination

- One side of the chest might not move as well (reduced expansion).
- The overlying chest wall may be hyper-resonant to percussion (louder and lower-pitched sounds than the low-pitched, hollow sounds that are elicited when tapping on a chest over normal lung tissue).
- The heart's apex beat may have moved!
- Breath sounds may be decreased or absent. This can be misleading in ventilated patients.

Investigations
- Chest X-ray (if there is time).

Why is pneumothorax more dangerous in mechanically ventilated patients?

A life-threatening *tension pneumothorax* may develop. Here, the 'tear' acts like a one-way valve; each inward breath 'pumps' more air out of the lung, but the 'valve' prevents it from getting back into the lung, so the situation gets steadily worse.

In a patient who is mechanically ventilated, the situation may deteriorate rapidly, as the pressures are different to those in a non-ventilated patient (a patient who is connected to a ventilator is having at least some of the air pushed into the lungs, whereas a person who is not being mechanically ventilated essentially 'sucks' air in). If prompt action is not taken, the patient may die.

Treatment of pneumothorax

If you are looking after a patient who has a pneumothorax, and you are not experienced in treating this condition, **call for more experienced help**.

If the patient is breathless and needs to stay in hospital:
- give high-flow oxygen (10–15 l/min via a mask with reservoir bag).

If the patient **is not** being mechanically ventilated:
- small pneumothorax (< 15% or < 2 cm rim on chest X-ray): observation and repeat chest X-rays
- larger pneumothorax: needle aspiration or chest drain.

If the patient **is** being mechanically ventilated:
- **extreme emergency** (low blood pressure, high heart rate, low oxygen levels, unable to ventilate, i.e. near death): **relieve the tension by inserting a large-bore intravenous cannula (14G) anteriorly through the second intercostal space in the midclavicular line**
- non-extreme emergency: insert an intercostal chest drain.

Technique for insertion of intercostal chest drain

- The patient should be placed in a supine or semi-recumbent position, with the affected side slightly elevated.
- Flex the patient's arm over their head or on their hip in order to improve access to the area.
- Clean the chest wall and prepare the area with sterile drapes (if there is time).
- The operator should wash their hands and wear a gown, mask and gloves (if there is time).
- Local anaesthetic should be administered to the proposed insertion site.
- Make a small skin incision over the proposed insertion site.
- The most common insertion site is the fifth intercostal space, in the anterior axillary line.
- A chest drain (tube) may be passed utilising a blunt dissection or a Seldinger technique (a description of this technique is beyond the scope of this chapter).
- The chest drain is usually passed up to the apex (top) of the chest wall to drain the pneumothorax.
- Secure the drain with a suture.
- Connect the external end of the drain to a special bottle with an underwater seal (so that air cannot be sucked back up into the space). Bubbles should appear in the water as the air escapes from the chest.
- Apply sterile dressing and tape around the insertion area.
- Review the patient's vital signs.
- Check the position of the chest drain with a chest X-ray.

Further reading

- Hinds CJ, Watson D. *Intensive Care: a concise textbook*, 3rd edn. Philadelphia, PA: Saunders Elsevier; 2008. 165–166.
- Henry M, Arnold T, Harvey J. BTS guidelines for the management of spontaneous pneumothorax. *Thorax*. 2003; **58 (Suppl. II):** ii39–52.

19

Cardiac arrhythmias

Peter Bunting, Dawn Soo and Mike Dickinson

Cardiac arrhythmias are common in sick patients in the critical care unit. They are classified according to their point of origin as supraventricular or ventricular, the dividing point being the atrio-ventricular node. They can also be classified according to heart rate as either tachycardias or bradycardias. The effects that they have on the cardiac output and blood pressure will determine whether or not the abnormal rhythm is life-threatening. Treatment of arrhythmias may be undertaken with some thought of diagnosis and appropriate treatment, but some arrhythmias are cardiac arrest rhythms and will require immediate treatment following the Advanced Life Support (ALS) principles of Airway, Breathing, Circulation. This chapter will assume that appropriate resuscitation is being undertaken with treatment of the abnormal rhythm.

Recognition of the abnormal rhythm is the first stage of treatment. Figure 19.1 illustrates a normal ECG, showing a P wave followed by a QRS complex and a T wave.

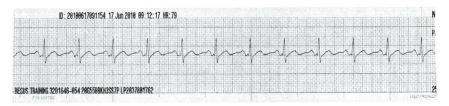

FIGURE 19.1

Supraventricular arrhythmias
Supraventricular tachycardia (SVT)

Supraventricular tachycardias can be divided into regular or irregular rhythms. Regular rhythms can be initiated from the sinoatrial (SA) node as sinus tachycardias, or the rhythm can be irregular due to atrial muscle contracting in an uncoordinated fashion, which is referred to as atrial fibrillation.

The most common arrhythmia on the ICU is atrial fibrillation (*see* Figure 19.2). This can be associated with hypovolaemia, electrolyte disturbance (most commonly low potassium and magnesium levels), acid–base abnormalities, cardiac ischaemia, valvular heart disease, and inflammatory processes (e.g. a middle lobe pneumonia causing irritation of the atrial muscle).

The rhythm is irregularly irregular, and if an arterial line is also *in situ* the height and width of each arterial pulse will vary. If the rate is slow, the cardiac output may not be compromised, but if the rate is fast the cardiac output may be reduced.

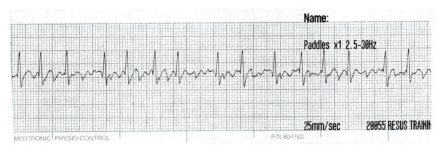

FIGURE 19.2

Treatment

A 12-lead ECG should be undertaken in all cases. Electrolytes, blood gases and acid–base status should also be measured. Low potassium and magnesium levels are common, and should be corrected. Acidic and hypoxic environments will not allow normal function of myocardial cells. Preload (volume status) also needs to be measured and corrected to allow normal atrial function. If blood pressure is low and cardiac output is life-threatening, electrical DC cardioversion is the treatment of choice. If the patient has a good cardiac output, drug therapy can be used. The first-line drug is amiodarone. Digoxin or beta-blockers may be used for rate control.

Atrial tachycardia

This may be physiological, as during exercise the heart rate may approach 180 beats/min. However, in the ICU it is always pathological. Narrow complex tachycardias are seen on ECG (*see* Figure 19.3).

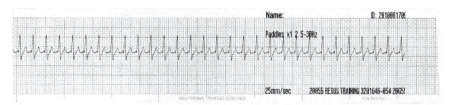

FIGURE 19.3

Treatment

Administration of adenosine will stop the action potential of the AV node and cause a few seconds of cardiac standstill, the heart then resuming in normal sinus rhythm. If the rhythm is atrial fibrillation (AF) or atrial flutter, the heart will not revert to sinus rhythm, as these rhythms are independent of the AV node.

Supraventricular bradycardias

The SA node can be ischaemic, and any critical illness can cause critical ischaemia and failure of the node. The result may be a sick sinus syndrome or failure to initiate the normal rhythm and a bradycardia.

Heart block

These rhythm abnormalities are due to the propagated action potential in the heart being prevented from progressing down the normal pathway. They are classified as first-, second- and third-degree block (*see* Figures 19.4 to 19.7). Second-degree block is further divided into Mobitz I (also called Wenkebach) and II.

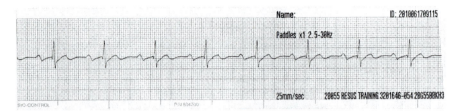

FIGURE 19.4

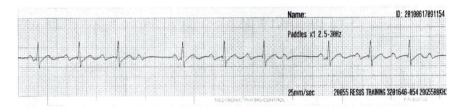

FIGURE 19.5

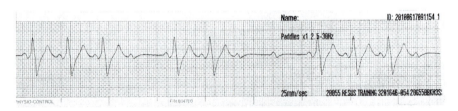

FIGURE 19.6

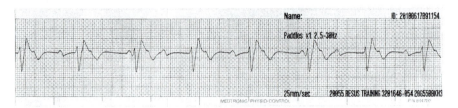

FIGURE 19.7

First-degree block is usually benign in itself, but can progress to higher degrees of block if provoked with drugs that decrease the activity of excitable tissue, such as anaesthetic and sedative agents and beta-blockers. Second-degree block can cause a fall in blood pressure due to missed beats, and as with first-degree block it can progress. Third-degree block means that no activity from the atria reaches the ventricular system, and the cells of the A-V node act as a pacemaker site for the ventricles. The inherent rate of contraction of these cells gives a heart rate of 40 beats/min. In most patients this means a drop in cardiac output of about 50%, which will be symptomatic.

Treatment
There are no drug treatments currently available, so the only treatment option is electrical pacing. The electrical signal is being blocked from progressing through the normal pathway, so external electricity is used to cause contraction of the ventricle. If the patient is symptomatic, external pacing pads should be used. If the patient is not symptomatic or is stable, transvenous pacing should be used.

Ventricular arrhythmias
Ventricular extrasystoles
Ventricular extrasystoles (*see* Figure 19.8) are common, and are of no consequence unless they are frequent (i.e. 1 in 2 or 3 beats), when they may cause a fall in cardiac output. If a run of extrasystoles occurs, this is ventricular tachycardia (*see* Figure 19.9). This can be slow, but more commonly it is fast, at 120 beats/min or faster. The patient may have a cardiac output or may be compromised.

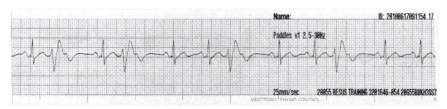

FIGURE 19.8

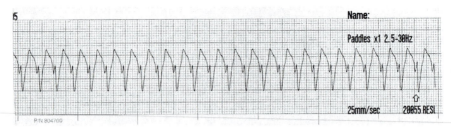

FIGURE 19.9

Treatment

The most effective treatment is urgent DC cardioversion. Drugs may be used as membrane stabilisers to prevent further episodes of this rhythm.

Ventricular fibrillation

This may be coarse (*see* Figure 19.10) or fine (*see* Figure 19.11). This is always a cardiac arrest rhythm, and it requires urgent resuscitation. A defibrillator will always be available on the critical care unit, but the principles of Airway, Breathing, Circulation must be followed to support the patient while the defibrillator is being prepared, to ensure that the myocardium is not hypoxic and acidotic, which would reduce the likelihood of successful defibrillation. Good CPR will also ensure some blood flow to vital organs and maintain the function of these organs.

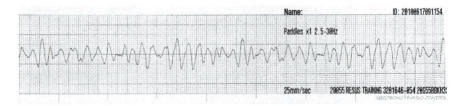

FIGURE 19.10

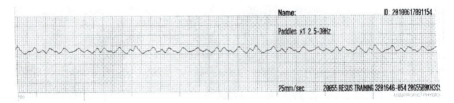

FIGURE 19.11

The drugs that are used to stabilise ventricular rhythms are membrane stabilisers such as lidocaine.

Asystole

Figure 19.12 shows asystole. Once again this is always a cardiac arrest rhythm, and CPR following BLS/ALS protocols should be started. Adrenaline should be administered to revert the rhythm to ventricular fibrillation, which can then be defibrillated to a normal rhythm.

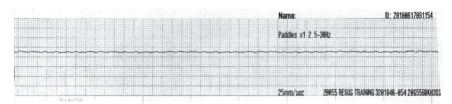

FIGURE 19.12

20

ICU delirium and the agitated patient

Nitin Arora

Definition of ICU delirium

Delirium has been defined as 'an acute, reversible, organic mental syndrome with disorders of attention and cognitive function, increased or decreased psychomotor activity and a disordered sleep-wake cycle.'[1]

ICU-related delirium has been referred to by various names in the past, including ICU confusion and ICU psychosis. It is a common condition, and affects 15–40% of critically ill patients.

It may present as:

- *hyperactive delirium* – agitated, paranoid patient (incidence around 2%)
- *hypoactive delirium* – withdrawn, quiet, paranoid patient (incidence around 45%)
- *mixed* – combination of hyperactive and hypoactive presentation (incidence around 53%).

The hyperactive form is usually well recognised, and the patient may be labelled as being 'agitated.' Such patients may show any of the following:

- continual movement (fidgeting, pulling at clothes, catheters or tubes, moving from side to side)

- disorientation
- failure to follow commands.

Risk factors for development of ICU delirium

Patient factors
- Elderly
- Comorbidities
- Pre-existing cognitive problems
- Hearing or vision impairment
- Alcoholism, smoking and substance abuse

Acute illness
- Acute respiratory distress syndrome (ARDS)
- Severe sepsis
- Multi-organ failure
- Drug overdose

Iatrogenic/environmental factors
- Sedative drug use
- Sleep deprivation
- Immobilisation
- Malnutrition

Why does delirium need to be prevented or treated?

Delirium is associated with increased length of ICU stay and increased morbidity and mortality.

Agitated delirious patients may harm themselves by pulling at invasive lines or catheters, and can even self-extubate. They are also at risk of falls and causing injury to members of staff.

Assessment of patients for delirium

Delirium screening tools appropriate for an ICU setting have been developed. The most commonly used are the Confusion Assessment Method for ICU (CAM-ICU) and the Intensive Care Delirium Screening Checklist

(ICDSC). The CAM-ICU is quick and simple to perform, and has excellent sensitivity and specificity.

It is easier to prevent delirium than to treat it. Delirium can be prevented by:

- avoiding deliriogenic medication (e.g. benzodiazepenes, barbiturates, drugs with antimuscarinic activity)
- psychological support and orientation (make sure that there is a visible clock, and have radio/TV news around the patient). Staff and family should try to communicate with the patient. Replace spectacles and hearing aids as soon as is practicable
- unambiguous environment, with a clear day–night cycle. Try to minimise noise and disturbance during sleeping hours (easier said than done on the ICU!)
- removing potential organic drivers for delirium (e.g. pain, hypoxia, hypercarbia, hypoglycaemia, metabolic or haemodynamic instability, withdrawal of drugs, etc.).

Treatment of delirium

Antipsychotics are the traditional mainstay of treatment of delirium, in response to the theory that delirium may be caused by a dopaminergic/muscarinic imbalance in the brain. Haloperidol is the most commonly used drug. Atypical antipsychotics such as olanzapine have also been shown to be effective, and have fewer side-effects.

Benzodiazepines worsen delirium and should be avoided except in patients with alcohol withdrawal, or to control acutely agitated patients who are a risk to themselves and to others.

A basic regime for management of delirium is suggested below.

Mild symptoms
Haloperidol 2–5 mg enterally three to four times daily, titrating to response, or olanzapine 5 mg enterally daily in patients who are unable to tolerate haloperidol (e.g. those with Parkinson's disease).

Moderate to severe symptoms
Haloperidol 0.5–10 mg intravenously (the dose is dependent on clinical parameters). Repeat as necessary. Continuous infusions of haloperidol

5–10 mg/hour may be required in extreme circumstances. Olanzapine 2.5–10 mg intramuscular injection, repeated after 2 hours if necessary in patients who are unable to tolerate haloperidol (e.g. those with Parkinson's disease).

Withdrawal delirium

This is generally treated with appropriate agents, such as benzodiazepines for ethanol, long-acting opioids for opioid dependence, clonidine for opioids or nicotine, nicotine patches for smoking cessation, etc.

How to deal with the agitated patient

- Correct any organic causes of the agitation.
- Try using IV or IM haloperidol. Olanzapine may be used if haloperidol is not tolerated.
- Judicious use of restraints such as bed rails or boxing gloves may help to prevent harm to both patient and staff.
- If the patient is dangerously agitated, short-acting sedative agents such as midazolam or propofol may be used, but only by staff who are trained in their use.
- There should be a low threshold for calling for senior advice.

Summary

Delirium is an under-recognised multi-factorial problem in ICU patients, and requires a multi-disciplinary approach for assessment, management and treatment.

Reference

1 British Journal of Anaesthesia. Editorial. *Br J Anaesth.* 2009; **103**: 2–5.

Further reading

- Ely EW, Margolin R, Francis J et al. Delirium in mechanically ventilated patients: validity and reliability of the Confusion Assessment Method for the Intensive Care Unit (CAM-ICU). *JAMA.* 2001; **286:** 2701–10.

- United Kingdom Clinical Pharmacy Association and Intensive Care Society. *UKCPA/ICS Guidelines for Detection, Prevention and Treatment of Delirium in Critically Ill Patients.* www.ukcpa.org/ukcpadocuments/6.pdf (accessed 17 January 2010).

21

Status epilepticus

Harry Chan

Patients who present with seizures may have a spectrum of different under-lying conditions. The involvement of the critical care team is frequently in response to seizures that are not responding to conventional treatments. This chapter reviews the recognition, causes, management and complica-tions of status epilepticus in adults.

Recognition

Convulsive status epilepticus is a medical emergency. It has been defined as any tonic–clonic seizure that lasts longer than 30 minutes, or the occur-rence of successive seizures without regaining consciousness for 30 minutes. The incidence is around 0.02% of the population, and the condition most commonly occurs in children and in patients with structural brain lesions. It has been reported to occur in 1 in 20 patients with established epilepsy. The associated overall mortality is around 20%. When tonic–clonic seizures last longer than around 30 minutes, autoregulation of cerebral blood flow is disrupted. After 60 minutes, there is an abrupt increase in mortality and an increased risk of irreversible brain injury. Prompt treatment reduces the severity of neurological injury from this potentially devastating condition.

Causes

There are many possible causes of status epilepticus. It may arise in someone with known idiopathic epilepsy, or it may be a new presentation in someone who is not known to be epileptic. In either case, there are a multitude of potential triggers, which may include metabolic, toxic or drug-related, vascular, acute or chronic structural brain conditions. It is very important to pursue the underlying cause, not only because it may affect initial management, but also because several underlying conditions warrant early treatment to prevent further morbidity.

Precipitants of seizures

These include the following:

- anti-epileptic drug withdrawal, drug interaction or toxicity
- alcohol withdrawal
- acute illness (e.g. sepsis)
- traumatic brain injury
- cerebrovascular accident
- encephalitis
- brain tumour
- electrolyte disturbances
- hypertensive emergencies.

Clues may be picked up during the history, examination and investigation of the patient. Relatives or witnesses can be an invaluable resource. Has the patient previously been diagnosed with epilepsy? A previous history indicates that a drug-related or chronic structural cause is more likely. Has the patient been unwell recently or was this an abrupt event? An abrupt, isolated event suggests a vascular cause. Is the patient taking any medications or recreational drugs, and have there been any changes in their prescription? The effectiveness of anti-epileptic drugs may be influenced by the addition of new medication. What is their alcohol consumption? Has there been a change in the pattern of drinking? On examination, what are the pupils like? Patients who have seizures typically have dilated, symmetrical, reactive pupils. Unequal and unreactive pupils suggest a structural brain lesion. Note the heart rate and blood pressure. During the early stages of a seizure the sympathetic nervous system is activated, resulting in a relative tachycardia and hypertension. In the later stages, hypotension may be apparent. Have there been any injuries as a result of the seizure? Are there signs of excessive alcohol consumption or chronic liver disease? Although this increases the likelihood of an alcohol-related seizure, bear in mind that these patients are also at risk of intracerebral bleeding and infections.

Management

Initial management should involve resuscitative measures and early control of seizures. Following the control of the seizure, the focus should be on identifying and treating any underlying precipitant and complications. Realistically, most patients with status epilepticus will require anaesthesia, intubation and ventilation in the first instance. This allows effective control of the situation and subsequent prompt investigation of the underlying cause.

Resuscitative measures

Airway

Place the patient on high-flow oxygen via a mask with a reservoir bag. If the mask is misting or the bag is deflating, this suggests patency of the airway. Patients with status epilepticus commonly have a partially obstructed airway as a result of their reduced conscious level. Oropharyngeal airways may be used but are commonly difficult to insert, as many of these patients have jaw rigidity and clenched teeth. An appropriately sized nasopharyngeal airway often helps to relieve the airway obstruction to some extent.

Cervical spine

Is there a possibility of neck injury? Patients who have fallen from a height of 2 metres or more, or who have had head injuries related to road traffic accidents, are at risk of neck injury. Consider cervical spine immobilisation if this is the case.

Breathing

During a tonic–clonic seizure, contraction of the chest wall and abdominal muscles results in restricted and shallow breathing. Uncorrected partial upper airway obstruction further reduces gas exchange. Generalised seizure activity also increases the metabolic rate. The overall result is less efficient breathing in the face of an increased oxygen demand. This predisposes to hypoxia and hypercarbia. The presence of vomitus on the patient and the presence of chest signs such as wheeze, crepitations or rhonchi suggest the possibility of aspiration of gastric contents. Be aware that chest signs may actually indicate the presence of acute pulmonary oedema secondary to left ventricular failure, particularly in the older patient. Arterial blood gases typically show a mixed respiratory and metabolic acidosis. If breathing is inadequate or if the patient remains significantly hypoxic (e.g. $SaO_2 < 90\%$ on 15 l/min reservoir mask) or hypercarbic (e.g. $PaCO_2 > 10\,kPa$), despite correction of any airway obstruction, consideration should be given to early intubation and mechanical ventilation.

Circulation

Establish intravenous access as soon as possible. This will allow the early administration of anticonvulsant drugs and intravenous fluids. Glucose and thiamine can be given if indicated. Once intravenous access has been established, blood should be sent off for urgent investigation (see below) if possible. An arterial blood gas analysis is useful to note the efficiency of gas exchange and the severity of the acidaemia. Patients who are convulsing are typically flushed, hypertensive and tachycardic. The presence of hypotension (i.e. systolic blood pressure < 90mmHg) in a patient with status epilepticus reflects a prolonged episode, and is associated with a worse outcome. Urgent fluid resuscitation is required, and vasopressors may be needed to ensure adequate cerebral perfusion.

Disability

Observe and record the convulsive movements of the patient. Be aware of diagnoses that may mimic status epilepticus, such as dissociative seizures (discussed later in this chapter). Tonic–clonic movements may become less pronounced as the duration of the seizure increases. Look at the pupils. Patients who are convulsing tend to have bilaterally dilated, reactive pupils. The presence of a fixed and dilated pupil suggests a structural brain lesion or intracerebral haemorrhage, and the patient is likely to need anaesthesia, intubation, ventilation and an urgent CT of the head. Measures to maintain an adequate cerebral perfusion pressure should be employed, by maintaining an adequate mean arterial pressure (e.g. 80–100 mmHg) and keeping the intra-cranial pressure as low as possible. The intracranial pressure can be reduced by keeping the head elevated more than 20° above the body, ensuring that the endotracheal tube ties are not restricting venous neck drainage, and also making sure that there is adequate oxygenation and a normal $PaCO_2$ (4–5 kPa).

Exposure
Perform a head-to-toe examination of the patient. Look for signs of head injury, tongue biting and limb injuries. The presence of purpura suggests the possibility of intracerebral bleeding. Record the tympanic temperature. The presence of a pyrexia does not necessarily indicate sepsis, as many patients with status epilepticus are moderately hyperthermic. Similarly, a leucocytosis is quite commonly observed after a seizure.

Glucose levels
An easily treatable cause of convulsions is hypoglycaemia. A blood glucose level can be measured rapidly with a glucometer or with certain blood gas machines. If the patient has significant hypoglycaemia (e.g. BM < 3), give intravenous glucose (e.g. 50 ml of 50% glucose).

Summary of initial resuscitative measures
1 Secure the airway/cervical spine stabilisation/oxygenation/with or without intubation.
2 Establish early intravenous access.
3 Administer anticonvulsants/IV fluids.
4 Send blood for analysis of the following: FBC, U&Es, glucose, calcium, magnesium, LFTs, clotting, arterial blood gases, anticonvulsant drug levels, toxicology (if suspected).
5 Establish monitoring (cardiac monitor, blood pressure, pulse oximetry, core temperature).
6 Consider the need for intravenous glucose if the patient is hypoglycaemic, or for thiamine (Pabrinex) if there is malnutrition and/or excessive alcohol consumption.

Anticonvulsant therapy
Most seizures self-terminate within 3 minutes and do not progress to status epilepticus or require anticonvulsant treatment. If a seizure lasts for more

than 3 minutes, anticonvulsant therapy should be administered, with a view to stopping the seizure as soon as possible. The longer the duration of a seizure, the more resistant it is to anticonvulsant therapy. The following is a guide to the pharmacological treatment of status epilepticus. Please note that specific guidelines may exist within different institutions, and where such guidelines exist they should be adhered to. Although organised into different stages according to the duration of status, the time frame is purely conceptual, and the key point is expedient management with control of the seizure. The bypassing of certain stages may be warranted depending on the level of clinical urgency.

Prehospital stage

In situations where intravenous access is not available or monitoring is limited, alternative routes of administration of benzodiazepines may be used. Diazepam 10–20mg PR may be given every 15 minutes. Midazolam 10mg buccal liquid is also effective.

Early status epilepticus (up to 30 minutes)

Lorazepam 0.1mg/kg IV (usually 4mg) given as a bolus is the initial drug of choice if intravenous access is available. It has a longer duration of action than either diazepam or midazolam. If seizures continue for more than 10 minutes, a second dose of lorazepam may be given.

Established status epilepticus (more than 30 minutes)

Phenytoin 15–18mg/kg as an IV infusion at a rate not exceeding 50mg/min should be commenced as a loading dose. This drug may be associated with significant cardiac arrhythmias and hypotension, so cardiac monitoring is essential. It is also highly immiscible with other drugs, and should be reconstituted in 0.9% saline and administered via a dedicated IV cannula. The prodrug, fosphenytoin, has advantages if it is available. It causes less phlebitis and hypotension, and is administered at a dose of 15–20mg phenytoin equivalents/kg at a higher maximum rate of 150mg/min.

An alternative to phenytoin at this stage of treatment is the barbiturate phenobarbitone. This may be given as an IV bolus of 10mg/kg at a rate of 100mg/min.

Refractory status epilepticus (more than 30–60 minutes)

These patients are at risk of irreversible brain damage, and it is vital to control the seizures immediately. General anaesthesia with thiopentone has been recommended as first-line treatment at this stage, and is highly effective. A loading dose of 3–5 mg/kg is given, followed by intubation and ventilation. Further boluses of 50–100 mg may be given every 2–3 minutes until the seizures are controlled. Skilled anaesthetic assistance is required, as the barbiturate causes profound cardiorespiratory depression.

The non-barbiturate general anaesthetic, propofol, has also been used effectively. Titrated to effect, and typically at a dose of 1–2 mg/kg, it has a similar rapid onset to thiopentone, and a more rapid offset. Again, considerable cardiorespiratory and CNS depression occurs, and hypotension may be pronounced.

Stabilisation and finding the precipitant

Once status epilepticus has been controlled, attention should be focused on stabilising the patient and establishing the underlying precipitant. If the patient is intubated, sedation will be necessary. A propofol (2–10 mg/kg/hour) or midazolam (0.05–0.5 mg/kg/hour after a loading dose of 0.1 mg/kg) infusion may be used for this purpose. Mechanical ventilation should be targeted to achieve a normal $PaCO_2$ of 4–5 kPa. Arterial cannulation and central venous access may be warranted, and the timing of these will depend on the cardiovascular stability of the patient. A nasogastric tube may be inserted and allows the drainage of gastric contents, thereby reducing the risk of aspiration. The use of intermediate- to long-acting muscle relaxants should be avoided if possible, as it hinders the recognition of further seizures.

Stabilisation should occur in tandem with arrangements to elucidate the cause of status epilepticus. In most cases, unless the precipitant is clear (e.g. anticonvulsant withdrawal in a patient with established epilepsy), imaging of the brain is required. This may be in the form of CT or MRI. Further investigation in the form of lumbar puncture and CSF sampling may be indicated if meningitis, encephalitis or subarachnoid haemorrhage is suspected. However, note that significant cerebral oedema or mass lesions may contraindicate this investigation, due to the risk of cerebral herniation. If severe sepsis or viral encephalitis is strongly suspected, early broad-spectrum antibiotics or antiviral therapy should be commenced as soon as possible.

Early referral to a specialist neurosurgical centre may be indicated when the neuroimaging results have been obtained.

Complications

Several complications may arise after status epilepticus, either as a result of the physiological impact on the body or as a result of treatment. They include the following:

- musculoskeletal complications (e.g. head injury, bone fractures)
- rhabdomyolysis and acute kidney injury
- metabolic acidosis and hyperthermia
- cerebral hypoxia
- tachyarrhythmias, hypertension and hypotension
- myocardial ischaemia
- pulmonary oedema
- pulmonary aspiration of gastric contents, acute respiratory distress syndrome (ARDS) and multi-organ failure.

Ongoing intensive care

Patients in whom seizures are controlled may be commenced on maintenance anticonvulsant therapy (e.g. phenytoin) in order to prevent seizure recurrence. Those with established epilepsy should have their usual anticonvulsants continued as soon as possible. Some patients may have seizures that are resistant to standard treatment. Such cases may be treated with infusions of thiopentone, propofol or midazolam. EEG monitoring is useful, and is recommended under such circumstances in order to monitor further epileptic activity and titrate anaesthetic doses. More specifically, anaesthetic doses are titrated primarily to cause suppression of epileptiform activity and secondarily to produce a 'burst suppression' pattern on the EEG. In situations where seizures still persist despite anaesthetic coma, the addition of other anticonvulsants such as topiramate and levetiracetam has been beneficial. Where patients are at risk of intracranial hypertension, ICP monitoring may be used to direct therapy and interventions.

Once seizure control has been maintained for a period of at least 12 hours, sedation may be slowly tapered off, with the aim of extubation where possible. Most patients with status epilepticus survive and have a relatively short stay in intensive care. The prognosis mainly depends on the reversibility of the underlying condition and the severity of any complications. There are two conditions that bear a resemblance to status epilepticus that may be under-recognised and worth mentioning. These are described below.

Pseudoseizures (dissociative seizures)

These are psychologically mediated episodes of altered behaviour or consciousness that may mimic a seizure. The patient may have an established history of epilepsy, and differentiation between a true epileptic seizure and a dissociative seizure can be difficult. If pseudoseizures are unrecognised, patients are invariably exposed to the iatrogenic risks associated with overmedication, drug toxicity, drug teratogenicity and intubation with mechanical ventilation in the setting of presumed status epilepticus. Dissociative seizures have no pathognomonic clinical features, but there are signs that are suggestive of the condition. Dissociative seizures tend to have a gradual onset, show a fluctuating degree of motor activity, last longer than 2 minutes, and there is an abrupt recovery. Resistance against eyelid opening, as well as violent limb movements, opisthotonus, pelvic thrusting and side-to-side head movements suggest the diagnosis. Pupillary reaction, corneal reflex and plantar responses are normal during a dissociative seizure. In challenging cases, the gold standard investigation of choice is video EEG telemetry, which allows EEG and video recording at the time of a seizure. Interestingly, the condition is thought to be an involuntary, trance-like state. Psychological support should be offered, and further management may include gradual withdrawal of anti-epileptic medication.

Non-convulsive status epilepticus

Some patients have ongoing electrical activity suggestive of seizures, but have minimal or no motor component reflecting seizure activity. This may present in an individual who remains comatose following generalised convulsive status epilepticus. However, it may also present with more subtle features, such as a change in behaviour or prolonged confusion after a seizure. A high index of suspicion and awareness of the condition are therefore needed. The diagnosis of non-convulsive status epilepticus (NCSE) can be difficult, and is reliant on EEG findings. There are different forms of

NCSE, and the response to anti-epileptic drugs can vary. The prognosis is also variable, depending mainly on the underlying condition, and is worst if the patient is in a coma after status epilepticus. Anti-epileptic treatment is usually warranted in NCSE, as electrographic seizures have the potential to cause further neuronal damage. Benzodiazepines, such as lorazepam and midazolam, have been used as first-line treatment. However, the urgency of treatment is not perceived to be as important as in convulsive status epilepticus.

Further reading

- Walker MC. Status epilepticus on the intensive care unit. *J Neurol*. 2003; **250:** 401–6.
- Walker MC. Status epilepticus: an evidence-based guide. *BMJ*. 2005; **331:** 673–7.
- Scottish Intercollegiate Guidelines Network. *Diagnosis and Management of Epilepsy in Adults: a national clinical guideline. SIGN Guideline No. 70.* Edinburgh: Scottish Intercollegiate Guidelines Network; 2003.
- Stokes T, Shaw EJ, Juarez-Garcia A *et al. Clinical Guidelines and Evidence Review for the Epilepsies: diagnosis and management in adults and children in primary and secondary care.* London: Royal College of General Practitioners; 2004.

22

Pneumonia

Huw Twamley

Community-acquired pneumonia (CAP)

This is defined by the British Thoracic Society as 'symptoms and signs consistent with a lower respiratory tract infection associated with new radiographic shadowing for which there is no other explanation.'

Organisms responsible

These include the following:

- *Streptococcus pneumoniae*
- *Haemophilus influenzae*
- *Legionella* spp.
- *Staphylococcus aureus*
- less commonly, *Moraxella catarrhalis*, Gram-negative enteric bacteria, *Mycoplasma*, *Klebsiella*.

Clinical findings and radiographic appearance do not reliably differentiate between the possible causative organisms.

The mortality of patients admitted to critical care in the UK has been found to be greater than 50% in some studies.

On admission to hospital, all patients with CAP should be assessed for severity of the condition. The most widely used scoring system is the CURB-65 score:

- **C**onfusion
- **U**rea > 7 mmol/l
- **R**espiratory rate > 30 breaths/min
- **B**lood pressure (systolic, < 90 mmHg; diastolic, < 60 mmHg)
- age > **65** years.

Each of these components, if present, scores 1 point. If a total score of ≥ 3 is obtained, the patient should be looked after in an intensive care area.

Consider ICU admission with or without intubation/ventilation if the patient has any of the following:

- severe CAP that is not responding rapidly to treatment
- persistent hypoxia
- progressive hypercapnia
- severe acidosis (pH 7.26)
- shock
- depressed consciousness.

Initial investigations

- Chest X-ray, arterial blood gas analysis, blood and sputum cultures.
- *Legionella* and pneumococcal urine antigen tests.

Initial therapy

- Antibiotics (see local guidelines):

  co-amoxiclav 1.2 g three times a day   clarithromycin 500 mg twice a day
  or
  cefuroxime 1.5 g three times a day   cefotaxime 1 g three times a day.

- Some areas use levofloxacin plus benzylpenicillin.
- Antibiotics can be modified depending on the culture results.
- The duration of treatment should be 10 days, or 14–21 days for *Legionella*, staphylococcal or Gram-negative enteric bacteria.
- Steroids are not useful in CAP.
- Ventilation should be used as indicated.

- Non-invasive ventilation has not been shown to be useful unless there is acute exacerbation of COPD.

Ventilator-associated pneumonia

- The incidence of this condition varies considerably depending on the diagnostic criteria.
- It is defined as pneumonia in a patient who has been intubated and ventilated, either at the time of or within 48 hours after the event.
- It increases mortality by approximately 30%, and it also increases the length of time on a ventilator and the length of stay on the critical care unit.
- It is probably caused by micro-aspiration from the oropharynx.

Diagnosis

Aim to differentiate between tracheobronchitis and true lower respiratory tract infection.

A diagnosis that is based on clinical findings may over-diagnose the condition. Clinical findings may be scored and amalgamated by using the clinical pulmonary infection score (CPIS), which scores for:

- tracheal secretions
- chest X-ray infiltrates
- temperature
- white cell count
- PaO_2/FiO_2 ratio.

The scores may be combined with a positive culture result.

Note that the threshold score for treatment may vary between centres.

Causative organisms

- Early onset (during first 4 days of admission): similar to community-acquired pneumonia.
- Late onset (more than 4 days after admission): Gram-positive organisms are more likely to be the cause. *Staphylococcus aureus*, *Pseudomonas* and *Klebsiella* are commonly isolated. The organisms are more likely to be resistant strains as they are hospital acquired.

Cultures

- Sputum samples are not a reliable way to identify organisms and make a diagnosis.
- Non-directed bronchi-alveolar lavage: 10 ml of saline are instilled into the trachea via an endotracheal or tracheostomy tube, and then suctioned in an aseptic manner. This technique may be as effective as bronchoscopic samples.
- Blind bronchial sampling: catheters are directed into the relevant lobes without the use of bronchoscopes.
- Bronchoscopic samples: this method is invasive and time-consuming, but allows deep sampling. It confirms the presence of infection through a differential white cell count of the sample and an organism count.

Prevention and risk reduction

The ventilator-associated pneumonia (VAP) prevention bundle seeks to reduce the incidence of VAP. Its components are as follows.

- Sedation to be reviewed and, if appropriate, stopped each day.
- All patients to be assessed for weaning and extubation each day.
- Avoid the supine position and aim to have the patient at least 30° head up.
- Use chlorhexidine as part of daily mouth care.
- Use subglottic secretion drainage in patients who are likely to be ventilated for more than 48 hours.

Other measures that may help reduce VAP incidence include the following.

- Adopt rigorous hand hygiene practices using alcohol gel.
- Avoid intubation (e.g. non-invasive ventilation).
- Use a LoTrach™ tube, which is designed to maintain a constant seal with cuff to reduce micro-aspiration.
- Maintain good cuff pressure. Even with non-specialised tubes this may reduce VAP.
- Ventilator circuit changes should take place weekly.
- Selective gut decontamination can be achieved by using a regime of prophylactic oral antibiotics to sterilise the gut. This may increase the levels of multi-resistant organisms.

Treatment

- Consult local guidelines.

- Tazobactam/piperacillin or ciprofloxacin are commonly used.
- If there is early onset as CAP, use co-amoxiclav.

Duration of antibiotics

- It may only be necessary to give antibiotics for 5 days. However, some experts recommend 7–10 days of treatment.
- The duration of treatment may need to be altered depending on the organism grown and its sensitivity to the antibiotic.
- Some centres use repeated daily bronchoscopic sampling, and if significant numbers of white cells are not found in the sample, the antibiotic is stopped.

Further reading

- British Thoracic Society. *BTS Guidelines for the Management of Community-Acquired Pneumonia in Adults.* London: British Thoracic Society.
- American Thoracic Society and Infectious Diseases Society of America. Guidelines for the management of adults with hospital-acquired, ventilator-associated and healthcare-associated pneumonia. *Am J Respir Crit Care Med.* 2005; **171:** 388–416.

23

Sepsis

Anita Jeh and Nitin Arora

Definitions

Sepsis can be viewed as a spectrum of disease that includes systemic inflammatory response syndrome (SIRS), sepsis, severe sepsis and septic shock.

SIRS is defined as the presence of two or more of the following:

- temperature > 38°C or < 36°C
- heart rate > 90 beats/min
- respiratory rate > 22 breaths/min
- white cell count > 12 000 cells/mm^3 or < 4000 cells/mm^3.

Sepsis is defined as SIRS with evidence of infection from a proven or suspected organism.

Severe sepsis occurs when organ dysfunction and hypoperfusion are present.

Septic shock is defined as sepsis associated with hypotension despite adequate fluid resuscitation, altered mental status and/or lactic acidosis.

Clinically, there is often a progression from SIRS to sepsis, to septic shock, to multi-organ dysfunction syndrome.

Common causes include pneumonia, urinary tract infection, meningitis, peritonitis, cholangitis, pancreatitis, abscess formation and cellulitis.

Sepsis can be complicated by acute respiratory distress syndrome (ARDS), acute kidney injury (AKI), disseminated intravascular coagulation (DIC), multiple organ failure, and death.

Signs and symptoms

Septic patients often present with altered mental status. If the latter is due to inadequate brain perfusion in sepsis it may commonly be manifested as restlessness, agitation or confusion.

On examination, patients are usually tachypnoeic, tachycardic, hypotensive, febrile (often with chills) or hypothermic. Hypothermia is more common in very young, elderly, debilitated and immunocompromised patients. There may be manifestations related to the cause of sepsis, such as pneumonia, urinary tract infection or peritonitis.

Patients with SIRS may have a bounding pulse, warm extremities, and rapid capillary refill due to peripheral vasodilatation, whereas those with severe sepsis and septic shock have a weak pulse, cool extremities, and slow capillary refill due to relative hypovolaemia caused by leaky capillaries.

Shock is often defined as low blood pressure, but it can exist despite a normal blood pressure, and conversely a low blood pressure may be compatible with adequate tissue perfusion.

Patients with sepsis are inappropriately dilated peripherally, and systemic vascular resistance (SVR) is severely decreased, which directly affects the blood pressure, as

$$MAP = CO \times SVR$$

where MAP is the mean arterial pressure, and CO is the cardiac output.

Low blood pressure in the presence of sepsis is related to low tissue perfusion and oxygenation, and the effects of low perfusion and oxygenation are manifested by a decreased Glasgow Coma Scale (GCS) score, reduced urine output and elevated lactate levels.

Cardiac output is normal or increased in septic shock, due to the maintenance of stroke volume and tachycardia, but the ejection fraction is decreased secondary to a reduction in contractility.

Parameters that are useful in the diagnosis and management of sepsis

- pH
- Lactate levels as an indicator of tissue hypoperfusion and hypoxia (which leads to anaerobic metabolism): a value of > 2 mmol/l is cause for concern, and a value of > 4 mmol/l is critical.
- Mean arterial pressure (MAP).
- End-organ perfusion, as indicated by measurements of urine output.
- Central venous pressure (CVP).
- Oxygen extraction (ScvO$_2$), which is a measure of the balance between oxygen delivery and consumption.

Sepsis is essentially a clinical diagnosis, and it can be confirmed by positive blood cultures. However, negative cultures are common.

Management and treatment

- ABCDE approach as in general emergency management.
- Management of severe sepsis, septic shock and/or lactate levels > 4 mmol/l is based on *Surviving Sepsis Campaign: international guidelines for management of severe sepsis and septic shock.*[1]

Initial resuscitation: goals during the first 6 hours

- CVP of 8–12 mmHg (12–15 mmHg in mechanically ventilated patients).
- MAP > 65 mmHg.
- Urine output > 0.5 ml/kg/hour.
- Central venous oxygen saturation > 70% or mixed venous oxygen saturation > 65%.

These goals can be achieved as follows:
- Measure serum lactate levels and obtain blood cultures prior to antibiotic administration (two or more blood cultures with at least one percutaneous sample). One blood culture from each vascular access device that is in place for more than 48 hours is needed.
- Administer a broad-spectrum IV antibiotic within the first hour of recognising severe sepsis or septic shock.

- Fluid therapy to treat hypotension and/or elevated lactate levels is imperative. Deliver initial challenges of 1000 ml of crystalloids or 300–500 ml of colloids over 30 minutes. Faster rates and larger volumes may be required depending on the patient's response to the fluid and the degree of tissue hypoperfusion. The rate of fluid administration may need to be reduced if cardiac filling pressures increase without a corresponding haemodynamic improvement.

- Fluid therapy may not be sufficient to achieve an MAP of > 65 mmHg, and the use of vasopressors such as noradrenaline or dopamine will help to achieve a higher MAP. Inotropic therapy with dobutamine is indicated in patients with elevated cardiac filling pressures and low cardiac output.

- The source of sepsis should be identified within the initial 6 hours of presentation, and imaging studies should be performed promptly to confirm and sample any source of infection. Source control measures should be implemented as soon as possible (e.g. abscess drainage, tissue debridement, and removal of suspected invasive lines or devices). The exception to this is infected pancreatic necrosis, where surgical intervention is best delayed.

Further goals and interventions to be implemented or considered during the first 24 hours from the onset of sepsis

- Control of glucose levels is also an important factor in resuscitation of patients with sepsis. Aim to keep blood glucose levels below 8.3 mmol/l, and monitor the levels 2- to 4-hourly.

- It is recommended that red blood cells are given when the haemoglobin concentration is < 7.0 g/dl in adults, and that platelets are administered when counts are < 5000/mm^3 in the absence of bleeding, or in the range 5000–30 000/mm^3 with a significant bleeding risk.

- Intravenous hydrocortisone can be considered for septic shock in adults where hypotension is not responding to adequate fluid resuscitation and vasopressors. The hydrocortisone dose should not exceed 300 mg/day. The use of corticosteroids to treat sepsis in the absence of shock is not recommended unless the patient's endocrine history warrants it.

- Activated protein C (APC) is believed to modulate coagulation and inflammation in severe sepsis. There is some evidence that APC improves the outcome in patients with multi-organ dysfunction if it is commenced within less than 48 hours.[2] Currently, APC is considered in adults with sepsis-induced organ dysfunction and a high risk of death (APACHE II > 25), or with multiple organ dysfunction in the absence of contraindications. However, it is strongly recommended that adults with severe sepsis and low risk of death (APACHE II < 20) do not receive APC.

In summary, the outcome in patients with sepsis improves significantly with rapid resuscitation to prevent prolonged tissue hypoxia, supportive measures, and early diagnosis and treatment of the underlying cause.

References

1 Dellinger RP, Levy MM, Carlet JM *et al.* Surviving Sepsis Campaign: international guidelines for management of severe sepsis and septic shock. *Intensive Care Med.* 2008; **34:** 17–60.
2 Bernard GR, Vincent JL, Laterre PF *et al.* for the PROWESS study group. Efficacy and safety of recombinant human activated protein C for severe sepsis. *N Engl J Med.* 2001; **344:** 699–709.

24

Acute respiratory distress syndrome

Craig Spencer

Acute respiratory distress syndrome (ARDS) is a syndrome of non-cardiogenic pulmonary oedema. It is characterised by diffuse alveolar and interstitial lung oedema, loss of surfactant, and alveolar flooding with a proteinaceous exudate that contains macrophages and neutrophils. This results in stiff, non-compliant lungs and hypoxaemia. The pathophysiology of the condition is complex, and is believed to be immunologically mediated by cytokines causing an inflammatory cascade and loss of capillary integrity. After 7–10 days a fibroproliferative stage develops, resulting in pulmonary fibrosis.

There should be a known precipitant for ARDS, which initiates the inflammatory response that causes lung injury. This may be a direct pulmonary cause, such as pneumonia, contusion, aspiration or smoke inhalation. Extra-pulmonary/systemic causes include sepsis, trauma, massive transfusion and pancreatitis.

Patients will present with signs of respiratory distress, including tachypnoea and cyanosis, often accompanied by signs of the precipitating condition.

Diagnosis

A similar less severe condition exists, known as acute lung injury (ALI), which shares many of the features of ARDS, but with less severe hypoxia. ALI may progress to ARDS.

American-European Consensus Conference (1994) definitions

- Acute onset.
- Bilateral infiltrates on chest X-ray.
- $PaO_2/FiO_2 < 200$ mmHg (c. 27 kPa) for ARDS; $PaO_2/FiO_2 < 300$ mmHg (c. 40 kPa) for ALI.
- No evidence of left atrial hypertension (including pulmonary artery occlusion pressure < 18 mmHg).

Treatment

This is directed at treating the precipitating cause of ARDS. Care should be taken to avoid secondary ventilator-associated lung injury (VALI) by over-distension or shearing forces applied to the alveoli. Ventilation should aim to avoid excessive tidal volume (volutrauma) or inspiratory pressure (baro-trauma) and repeated alveolar collapse (atelectrauma). Great care should be taken with regard to the prevention and early detection and treatment of nosocomial infection. Ventilation practice in ARDS changed significantly following the presentation of the landmark ARDSnet paper in 2000 and the introduction of low tidal volume ventilation.

Ventilation strategies

- There are reports of successful management of ARDS with non-invasive ventilation (NIV). The failure rate is high (around 70%), especially in the presence of severe hypoxia, metabolic acidosis and especially shock.
- Intubation and ventilation are the mainstay of supportive therapy, with the aim of avoiding hypoxia, excessive hypercapnia and VALI.
- Aim for tidal volumes of 6 ml/kg of ideal body weight (IBW), which is based on gender and height. Male IBW = 50 kg + 0.91 (cm of height – 152.4). Female IBW = 45.5 kg + 0.91 (cm of height – 152.4).
- Aim for a plateau pressure of 30 cmH$_2$O or less. It is unclear whether it is most important to avoid excessive pressure or excessive volume.

- Permissive hypercapnia may be considered. With low tidal volumes, hypercapnia is almost inevitable. A respiratory acidosis is usually tolerated down to around pH 7.2. Below this level the options include increasing the respiratory rate (with a risk of reducing the expiratory time and 'breath stacking'), giving IV sodium bicarbonate (which may cause intracellular acidosis), or relaxing the tidal volume limit to 7 or 8 ml/kg.

- Open lung ventilation involves the use of positive end-expiratory pressure (PEEP) to keep recruited alveoli open, avoid atelectrauma and improve oxygenation. In patients with ARDS the lung is not homogenous, and excessive PEEP risks over-distension in less affected parts, as well as cardiovascular effects such as reduced venous return with high intra-thoracic pressure. Selecting the right level of PEEP is difficult. However, a commonly used scale of 5–20 cmH$_2$O of PEEP that increases with FiO$_2$ is a good starting point.

- Inverse ratio ventilation. A physiological inspiratory/expiratory time ratio (I:E ratio) is 1:2, to allow time for passive expiration of carbon dioxide. At a high FiO$_2$, increasing the inspiratory time or even reversing the ratio from 1:2 to 2:1 gives extra time for inspiratory flow to redistribute to alveoli that are difficult to recruit. It may increase hypercapnia by reducing the time for passive carbon dioxide excretion.

- Prone ventilation. The prone position offers better ventilation/ perfusion matching and less lung base compression by the abdomen. The chest and pelvis should be supported to allow abdominal movement with ventilation. There is a risk of displacement of the airway and lines, and of facial pressure sores. Trials have tended to find a significant improvement in oxygenation in around 70% of patients (referred to as responders, as compared with non-responders), especially with prolonged prone periods of up to 20 hours/day. However, no trial has found a significant mortality benefit. Prone ventilation is often used a rescue or holding therapy as a patient approaches the need for FiO$_2$ of 1.0.

- High-frequency oscillation ventilation (HFOV). This uses a specialised ventilator to deliver small tidal volumes (around 100 ml) at very high respiratory rates (3–15 breaths/second). Tidal volumes are often less than lung dead space, and gas transfer is thought to take place by convective streaming. It is an extreme form of open lung ventilation, and has been used as a rescue therapy. A large multi-centre controlled trial is ongoing.

Sedation

Patients may need to be heavily sedated in order to tolerate relatively non-physiological ventilation strategies for non-compliant lungs, especially in the prone position. It may be necessary to abolish all patient effort in the early stages. Non-depolarising neuromuscular blockers (e.g. atracurium) may improve lung compliance in this group, but their use makes heavy sedation mandatory. Sedation is best titrated to a prescribed sedation score, such as the Richmond Agitation Sedation Scale (RASS). As lung mechanics improve, daily sedation holds can be used to enable spontaneous patient effort.

Other therapies

- Extracorporeal membrane oxygenation (ECMO) is a highly specialised therapy similar to cardiopulmonary bypass for cardiac surgery. The extracorporeal circuit adds oxygen and removes carbon dioxide, and requires anticoagulation. The recent CESAR trial showed a mortality benefit with transfer of patients with ARDS of less than 7 days' duration to a specialist centre (Glenfield Hospital, Leicester).
- Pulmonary vasodilators. Nitric oxide, when inhaled at concentrations of up to 40 ppm, crosses the alveoli in ventilated parts of the lung, causing local vasodilation and improved ventilation–perfusion matching and oxygenation. As with prone ventilation (see above), there are responders and non-responders to this approach. Nitric oxide is only rarely used as a rescue therapy, and no mortality benefit has been demonstrated. A similar approach has been attempted with the prostaglandin epoprostenol.
- Restrictive fluid therapy. Increased extravascular lung water is associated with increased mortality and prolonged respiratory weaning. A restrictive fluid administration regime, including the use of diuretics, that aims for an even fluid balance at 7 days post onset is associated with improved oxygenation and reduced time on a ventilator (but not reduced mortality), without increasing the need for renal replacement therapy.
- Steroids. Multiple trials have investigated whether the use of steroids may be beneficial, particularly in reducing the fibroproliferative stage

of ARDS between 7 and 14 days post onset. The evidence is mixed, as is practice.

Outcome

The outcome is dependent on the precipitant pathology. ARDS with an extra-pulmonary cause (e.g. sepsis) is associated with a higher mortality rate than is ARDS with a pulmonary cause that reflects multi-organ involvement. The mortality rate was around 60% when the condition was first described, it had fallen to about 40% by around 2000, and it fell again to 31% with the advent of 'ARDSnet ventilation.' Very few patients actually die of hypoxia, but rather it is the underlying precipitant, or complications such as infection, that lead to their death. Survivors often have some pulmonary fibrosis and reduced lung diffusing capacity, resulting in some functional respiratory impairment. A significant proportion of survivors may have no impairment at all.

Further reading

- Acute Respiratory Distress Syndrome Network. Ventilation with lower tidal volumes as compared with traditional tidal volumes for acute lung injury and the acute respiratory distress syndrome. *N Engl J Med*. 2000; **342**: 1301–8.

25

Acute renal failure in intensive care (acute kidney injury)

Nitin Arora and Shondipon Laha

> 'Mr Jones in Bed 12 has only passed 15 ml of urine in the last 3 hours. What do you want us to do?'

This is one of the commonest questions you are likely to be asked in intensive care on a night shift. Other specialties think that we are obsessed with urine output – and they are right!

There are two main categories of renal failure, namely acute and chronic. We predominantly see cases of acute renal failure, which occasionally evolve into the chronic category.

Renal failure affects a number of patients in intensive care, and is associated with significant morbidity and mortality. The prognosis is worse when renal failure occurs as part of multi-organ failure (the mortality rate exceeds 60% if renal replacement therapy is required).

Causes of renal failure

Acute renal failure on the intensive care unit is generally multi-factorial in origin. The causes can be divided into the following categories.

Pre-renal causes (generally due to poor renal perfusion)
- Volume depletion
- Severe hypotension
- Reduced cardiac output
- Renovascular disease (e.g. renal artery stenosis)

Renal causes
- Toxaemia (sepsis, iatrogenic causes, rhabdomyolysis)
- Hypoxia (sepsis, ARDS, cardiogenic shock)
- Vascular (Wegener's granulomatosis, atherosclerosis)
- Pre-existing glomerulonephritis

Post-renal causes (generally obstructive, and unlikely to be a major cause on the ICU)
- Blocked urinary catheter
- Enlarged prostate
- Increased abdominal pressure (compartment syndrome)
- Malignancy

Diagnosis of acute renal failure/acute kidney injury (AKI)

This is diagnosed on the basis of history and biochemical investigations. The following should be present:
- abrupt onset (less than 48 hours)
- deterioration of kidney function characterised by a rise in serum creatinine concentration (> 50% from baseline level, or an increase of 25 micromol/l)) and oliguria (< 0.5 ml/kg/hour for more than 6 hours).

Staging

The different stages of acute kidney injury (AKI) have been defined as RIFLE:
- **R**isk of AKI: a rise in serum creatinine concentration by > 50% from baseline, or urine output of < 0.5 ml/kg/hour for 6 hours.
- **I**njury: a rise in serum creatinine concentration by > 100% from baseline, or urine output of < 0.5 ml/kg/hour for more than 12 hours.

- Failure: a rise in serum creatinine concentration by 300% from baseline, or an increase by > 350 micromol/l, or urine output of < 0.3 ml/kg/hour for 24 hours or anuria for 12 hours.
- Loss: persistent loss of kidney function for 4 weeks.
- End-stage renal disease: loss of kidney function for more than 3 months.

Prevention of renal failure

There is no easy answer, but being aware of the risk factors and of the condition is the first step.

Investigations

Blood tests

- Urea and creatinine. Definitive levels that indicate renal failure are very unreliable, but an increasing trend in both is highly suggestive of the condition. If the ratio of urea to creatinine rises, this suggests a pre-renal cause.
- Potassium. Acute renal failure can often cause raised potassium levels (which may also be reflected by the ECG).
- Haemoglobin. An increase in haemoglobin and haematocrit suggests very concentrated blood and dehydration.

Blood gas analysis

- Increasing negative base excess, acidosis and rising lactate levels are all suggestive of possible renal failure causing metabolic acidosis.

Creatinine clearance

- Creatinine is an inert substance that is predominantly filtered by the glomerulus. It has a relatively constant plasma rate, and is routinely measured. Its clearance allows an approximation of glomerular filtration rate (GFR), but may be approximately 10% above actual GFR (due to not recognising the component of secreted creatinine).
- This is normally measured over a 24-hour period, but many units will measure it over 6 hours, providing a quicker but less accurate result.

Urine analysis
- This is undertaken for protein, blood, urinary sodium, osmolality, microscopy and culture.

Other investigations
- Other investigations, including radiography, should be guided by clinical suspicion of the cause.

Treatment of acute renal failure
Initial management: the first 6 hours
Remember your ABC
- Make sure that the airway is patent.
- Give 100% oxygen until the patient is in a stable environment and their respiratory history can be assessed.
- Make sure that there is adequate large-bore venous access. Does the patient appear clinically hypovolaemic? If so, give a bolus of fluid (crystalloid or colloid).
- Treat hyperkalaemia with calcium gluconate or an insulin/dextrose regime (there is normally a hospital protocol for this).

Lines
Often these patients will need a central venous catheter for assessing fluid status and for vasopressor support if required. An arterial line may also be needed. These patients should have a urinary catheter *in situ*, and urine output should be measured hourly.

Drugs
Diuretics (e.g. furosemide) are occasionally used once the patient is well hydrated to induce diuresis (but be wary about this, as it may cause further renal damage).

Sodium bicarbonate
- This is occasionally used as a temporary holding measure to correct a metabolic acidosis.
- Do not use it without seeking senior advice.
- Stop or minimise nephrotoxic drugs if possible.

Renal replacement therapy after the initial management

Renal replacement therapy (RRT) is the treatment of established renal failure that has not responded to the above initial management measures. Major indications for renal replacement therapy are as follows:

- fluid overload leading to pulmonary oedema that is not responding to diuretics
- hyperkalaemia that is unresponsive to medical management
- severe metabolic acidosis
- oliguria or anuria
- rising urea and creatinine levels
- drug overdose with a substance that is amenable to removal by dialysis.

Modes of renal replacement therapy

Renal replacement therapy seeks to artificially mimic the excretory function of the kidney. The feature shared by all of the methods is the use of a semi-permeable membrane for filtration.

There are various modes of delivery of renal replacement therapy, which can be summarised as follows:

- **Peritoneal dialysis.** The peritoneum acts as the semi-permeable membrane. Dialysis fluid is infused into the peritoneal cavity by means of a peritoneal catheter, is allowed to equilibrate with the body, and is then replaced after a few hours. This is a slow method and it does not work well on the ICU, mainly because of low efficiency, poor splanchnic circulation in the critically ill patient, and the need for a peritoneal catheter, which is a potential focus for infection and cannot be placed after, for instance, a laparotomy.
- **Haemodialysis.** This is a form of intermittent renal replacement therapy. Blood is drawn out of the body either through a large-bore double-lumen intravascular catheter or via needles inserted in an arteriovenous fistula, and is passed through an extracorporeal circuit, separated from the dialysate fluid by a semi-permeable membrane. Solutes, including urea and creatinine, are drawn out by osmosis across a concentration gradient. This is a rapid, highly efficient process, and it is the mainstay of chronic renal replacement in an outpatient setting. However, it is not commonly used on the ICU because it has the potential to cause more haemodynamic instability than haemofiltration.

- **Haemofiltration.** This is a convective process that uses a dialysis catheter and an extracorporeal circuit (similar to haemodialysis). An ultrafiltrate is produced from the blood using hydrostatic pressure that drives fluid and solutes across the membrane (similar to glomerular filtration). The ultrafiltrate is discarded and replaced by isotonic fluid. There is evidence that an ultrafiltration rate of 35 ml/kg/hour is associated with better outcomes. Haemofiltration is a slower process than haemodialysis, and often continues for hours or days. It generally has more cardiovascular stability, and is the preferred mode of renal replacement therapy in the UK. Modern haemofiltration is almost always continuous veno-venous haemofiltration (CVVH), although continuous arterio-venous haemofiltration (CAVH) has been used in the past.
- **Haemodiafiltration.** This combines the elements of haemodialysis and haemofiltration.

Problems with renal replacement therapy
- **Vascular access problems.** These include difficulty in obtaining good central access, or high access pressures even with central access that may necessitate a change of dialysis/haemofilter central venous catheter.
- **Need for anticoagulation.** Blood flowing through an extracorporeal circuit can trigger the clotting pathways, causing a loss of blood that is already in the circuit, and also necessitating replacement of an expensive circuit. The anticoagulant that is generally used is heparin, typically at 500–2000 units/hour, although prostacyclin may also be used. Patients who are coagulopathic may not require anticoagulation.
- **Air embolism.** This is uncommon with newer machines which have sophisticated air entrapment alarms.
- **Haemorrhage.** This may occur when obtaining vascular access, or it may be caused by a circuit disconnection.
- **Drug pharmacokinetics.** In patients on renal replacement therapy these can be very complex, and they differ from those for patients who are not on renal replacement. The dose and frequency of administration also differ between haemodialysis and haemofiltration. If in doubt, seek expert advice from the renal physicians, renal drug handbook or a renal pharmacist.

Long-term prognosis

Nearly two-thirds of patients with acute renal failure who survive to discharge will regain most of their renal function. However, around 15–30% require continuing renal replacement therapy after discharge from the unit, so they must be referred to, and managed jointly with, renal physicians.

Further reading

- Ronco C, Bellomo R, Homel P *et al*. Effects of different doses in continuous veno-venous haemofiltration on outcomes of acute renal failure: a prospective randomised trial. *Lancet*. 2000; **356:** 26–30.
- Acute Dialysis Quality Initiative: www.adqi.net
- Kellum JA, Bellomo R, Ronco C. Definition and classification of acute kidney injury. *Nephron Clin Pract*. 2008; **109:** c182–7.
- Intensive Care Society. *Standards and Recommendations for the Provision of Renal Replacement Therapy on Intensive Care Units in the United Kingdom*. London: Intensive Care Society; 2009.

26

Hepatic failure

Mark Pugh

Introduction

Primary acute liver failure is a relatively rare reason for admission to critical care units in the UK. Unfortunately, acute decompensation against a background of chronic liver disease is all too common (most commonly secondary to alcohol and, increasingly, hepatitis C). This chapter will address normal liver function, the causes of acute liver failure, how to evaluate liver function clinically and biochemically, and subsequent management and prognosis.

Normal liver function

The major functions of the liver are as follows:

- metabolism of fat, protein (synthesis, and deamination to urea) and carbohydrate (glucose synthesis, glucose storage in the form of glycogen, and glucose production from other substrates via the process of gluconeogenesis)
- production and breakdown of hormones
- removal of toxins, and conversion to less harmful metabolites (this includes drug metabolism)

- breakdown of red blood cells (and production of bile)
- synthesis of plasma proteins, albumin and clotting factors
- storage of vitamins A, D and B_{12}
- storage of essential minerals (iron and copper)
- immune function, including removal of bacteria and antigens.

Causes of acute liver failure

Toxins
- Paracetamol
- Antibiotics, anti-TB drugs, anti-epileptics, many other common drugs
- Cocaine, ecstasy
- Toadstools (classically death cap)

Infection
- Hepatitis A and B (but not usually C)
- Cytomegalovirus (CMV) and Epstein–Barr virus (EBV)

Other
- Fatty liver of pregnancy and HELLP syndrome
- Ischaemia (prolonged hypotension, heart failure)
- Decompensation of long-standing problems, such as Wilson's disease, haemochromatosis and alcohol abuse. Strictly speaking, this is acute chronic liver failure.

Assessment of liver function

Clinical assessment
- Symptoms and signs in acute liver failure can often be absent or confusing.
- Onset of jaundice and altered mental status should always raise the possibility of acute liver dysfunction.
- In patients with decompensated chronic liver disease the diagnosis is often more obvious, with jaundice, encephalopathy, spider naevi, ascites and variceal haemorrhage often being features at presentation.

Biochemical assessment

- Traditional 'liver function tests' (LFTs) are a complete misnomer – they tell you very little about the synthetic function of the liver (i.e. how well it is working). They may give clues to the cause of dysfunction. For example, elevated transaminases indicate a cellular problem (e.g. toxin, infection, ischaemia), whereas elevated alkaline phosphatase and gamma-glutamyl transferase (GGT) indicate a cholestatic picture (e.g. drugs, gallstones, obstruction).
- Synthetic tests:
  - **Prothrombin time (PT).** Prolongation of PT indicates that the liver is simply not producing enough clotting factors. **Do not correct prolonged PT unless there is life-threatening haemorrhage**, as it is an essential marker of progress and prognosis.
  - **Albumin.** This is a marker of protein synthesis, which can be low in patients with long-standing disease and malnutrition.
  - **Lactate.** Ordinarily the liver rapidly consumes lactate as a substrate for the production of energy and glucose. Elevated lactate levels are a marker of liver dysfunction.
  - **Glucose.** The liver needs to be 'on its knees' before it ceases to produce adequate amounts of glucose. Low blood glucose levels should be suspected and treated in all cases.
  - **Ammonia.** Protein is normally broken down in the liver, and the harmful ammonia-containing group is conveniently converted to urea for excretion by the kidneys. However, in liver failure this does not happen, and ammonia levels are consequently raised. They are believed to contribute to the development of encephalopathy.

Management of liver failure

The management of liver failure is similar to that of most other conditions. Suspect, diagnose, support and arrange definitive treatment where possible.

Suspect

- The presentation is not always obvious. Any history of onset of jaundice accompanied by confusion should raise suspicion.
- Obtain a clear history. Ask about medications, alcohol consumption,

the possibility of overdose, use of recreational drugs, IV drug usage, foreign travel, sexual history and family history (e.g. Wilson's disease).
- Perform a focused examination (encephalopathy, flap, skin, abdomen, ascites, etc.).

Diagnose
- Screen for hepatitis A, B, C and E.
- Screen for Wilson's disease and alpha-1 antitrypsin deficiency.
- Measure paracetamol levels in all patients.
- Perform the following investigations: baseline FBC, U&Es, LFTs and clotting factors.
- Perform relevant imaging (USS, CT, and also echocardiography if heart failure is the suspected cause).
- Ask for the help of a gastroenterologist with an interest in this field.

Support
- Airway, Breathing, Circulation, Disability. If the Glasgow Coma Scale (GCS) score is < 8, consider the need for airway protection.
- A, B, C, **D, E, F, G: D**on't **E**ver **F**orget **G**lucose. Monitor glucose levels closely, and correct them as necessary.
- Provide an appropriate level of care (HDU or ICU).
- Give N-acetylcysteine in all cases of paracetamol overdose, even if presentation is delayed. If the patient is at high risk, err on the side of treatment, even if the algorithm is equivocal.
- Give lactulose. This reduces the enterohepatic circulation of ammonia-containing compounds.
- Nutrition.
- Monitor synthetic function (INR), acid–base balance and renal function at regular intervals.
- **Do not correct the INR unless there is life-threatening haemorrhage**, because it is the most useful prognostic factor.
- Give vitamin replacement (especially thiamine/vitamin B complex in alcoholics).
- Treat infection aggressively.

Arrange definitive treatment
- Treat the cause where appropriate.

- For all patients who present with severe acute liver failure and who do not respond to simple treatment, seek advice from the Regional Liver Unit at the earliest opportunity, as your patient may require or be a suitable candidate for a liver transplant.
- Ordinarily, patients with an aetiology of chronic alcohol abuse would not be considered for a liver transplant unless they had been abstinent for the previous 6 months.
- The King's College criteria are the most widely used in the UK for assessment of the suitability of patients for liver transplantation (see reference below).

Prognosis

- Patients with acute liver failure who meet the criteria for liver transplantation have greater than 80% mortality without transplantation.
- With transplantation, 5-year survival rates are greater than 70%, and continue to improve.
- Patients with acute decompensation of alcoholic liver disease have an overall poor prognosis. This raises ethical issues with regard to their admission to critical care, particularly if they have had an episode of decompensation previously, but are continuing to drink despite advice to abstain.

Conclusions

Acute liver failure is relatively uncommon. Early recognition, appropriate resuscitation and early referral to a regional liver unit are in the patient's best interest.

Further reading

- O'Grady JG, Alexander GJ, Hayllar KM *et al*. Early indicators of prognosis in fulminant hepatic failure. *Gastroenterology*. 1989; **97:** 439–45.

27

Subarachnoid haemorrhage

Ian Donaldson

Definition

A subarachnoid haemorrhage (SAH) is defined as bleeding into the space between the arachnoid mater and the pia mater surrounding the brain.

Incidence

- Spontaneous haemorrhage has an incidence of approximately 5 patients per 100 000 patient years.
- It is twice as common in women as in men.
- It affects all age groups, but is commonest in the 50–65 years age range.

Mortality

- Approximately 50% of patients will not survive, and often they do not survive the initial event.
- One-third of survivors may remain dependent.

Risk factors

- Smoking
- Alcohol abuse
- Hypertension
- Family history
- Hereditary diseases (e.g. polycystic kidneys, connective tissue disorders)
- Anticoagulants and antiplatelet therapy probably do not increase the incidence of aneurysmal rupture, but will increase the severity of the condition if rupture occurs.

Presentation

- Patients present with a variety of symptoms and signs, ranging from a mild headache to sudden collapse and death.
- Classically there is sudden onset of a very severe occipital headache associated with nausea and vomiting.
- Photophobia and visual disturbance occur.
- Around 50% of patients will develop confusion, altered level of consciousness or focal neurology, which may improve quickly.
- Around 10% of patients will develop seizures.

Diagnosis

- A history and physical examination should be undertaken.
- The findings often include hypertension and tachycardia.
- Assess neck stiffness and check focal neurology, including cranial nerve palsies.

Investigations

- A non-contrast CT scan is the investigation of choice, as it identifies most cases.
- A normal CT scan with strong clinical suspicion should be followed by lumbar puncture after 12 hours. Xanthochromia confirms the diagnosis (yellow-stained CSF, due to the formation of bilirubin as a result of red cells being broken down).

Classification of SAH

The World Federation of Neurological Surgeons classifies patients with SAH according to the Glasgow Coma Scale (GCS) and the presence or absence of focal motor neurological deficit.

TABLE 27.1 Classification of patients with SAH

GCS SCORE	FOCAL MOTOR DEFICIT	GRADE
15	No	1
13–14	No	2
13–14	Yes	3
7–12	Yes or no	4
3–6	Yes or no	5

Survival rates may exceed 70% for good grades, but may be as low as 20% for poorer grades.

Causes

- SAH is classified as traumatic or non-traumatic.
- It may be difficult to distinguish between these categories after a 'collapse.' In such cases, CT appearance and the distribution of blood on the scan may aid classification.
- Around 85% of spontaneous bleeds occur from a cerebral aneurysm on or near the circle of Willis.
- Around 10% are non-aneurysmal, and no cause is found.
- Around 5% are due to rare conditions such as arteriovenous malformations, tumour, drug abuse and coagulopathy.

Complications

Immediate complications

- 'Catecholamine storm' occurs at the time of SAH, resulting in severe hypertension and systemic complications.
- Cardiac arrest, dysrhythmia, myocardial infarction or cardiogenic pulmonary oedema may occur.

- Virtually all ECG changes have been described, and they may or may not be ischaemic in origin.
- Respiratory failure, including aspiration and neurogenic pulmonary oedema.
- Seizures.
- Raised intracranial pressure (ICP) due to haematoma or hydrocephalus (which may develop over several days) may require an external ventricular drain (EVD).
- Delayed ischaemic deficit due to vasospasm may cause focal neurological deficit or a generalised reduction in conscious level.

Other complications
- Rebleeding. If untreated, as many as 40% of cases will rebleed in the 4 weeks after presentation (up to 5% in the first 24 hours).

Management
- Initial management consists of basic resuscitation.
- The aim is to prevent and treat immediate complications, reduce the likelihood of rebleeding by treating the source of the bleed, and reduce the incidence and severity of vasospasm.
- Adequate hydration is essential. Non-glucose crystalloids are preferred.
- Patients' blood pressure, temperature, arterial oxygen saturation and carbon dioxide should all be maintained within normal limits.
- Analgesics may help to control blood pressure, and beta-blockers or labetalol may be useful.
- Care should be taken with aggressive blood pressure control in patients with raised intracerebral pressure (hydrocephalus or haematoma), and this problem should be addressed first.
- Glucose control is important.
- Patients with altered levels of consciousness and/or seizures may require sedation and intubation or ventilation.
- It is essential to avoid any surges in blood pressure associated with intubation, in order to reduce the likelihood of rebleeding.
- All patients with suspected aneurysmal subarachnoid haemorrhage should be given nimodipine orally or via a nasogastric tube for 21 days post bleeding.

- An intravenous infusion should be given if the oral route is not available (hypotension is not uncommon, and usually responds to fluids).

Investigations

Initial investigations should include the following:
- full blood count
- urea and electrolytes, glucose, magnesium, bone and liver profile
- ECG
- other investigations as clinically indicated (chest X-ray, arterial blood gas analysis and troponin T test are commonly required)
- non-contrast CT scan once the patient is stable.

Discussion with neurosciences centre

- All patients with SAH should be discussed urgently with a neurosciences centre to plan further investigations and management.
- Cerebral angiography or CT angiography may be required.
- Insertion of an EVD may be required for management of hydrocephalus.
- Evacuation of an intracerebral haematoma and clipping of an aneurysm may be required urgently for some patients.
- Up to 95% of patients with aneurysmal disease will be suitable for endovascular coiling, which is normally performed within 24–48 hours of admission if possible.

Post-operative management

- Following definitive treatment of the source of bleeding, most patients will require a period of critical care.
- Good 'basic' critical care is essential.
- Ongoing management of complications is required.
- Specific management of delayed ischaemic deficit due to vasospasm can be implemented.
- Diagnosis can be assisted by serial transcranial Doppler monitoring.

- Triple-H therapy (hypertension, hypervolaemia and haemodilution) is commonly instituted.
- Specific radiological intervention, balloon angioplasty or intra-arterial nimodipine infusion also have a role.

28

Acute severe asthma

Huw Twamley

Management of asthma depends on initial assessment of the severity of the current episode, together with the identification of risk factors for near-fatal and fatal asthma.

Initial assessment

Danger signs in the history

The history should aim to identify the following factors, all of which increase the likelihood of progression to near-fatal or fatal asthma:

- background of severe asthma:
  - previous near-fatal asthma
  - previous ventilation
  - previous admission for asthma
  - patient requires three or more asthma medications
  - repeated attendance at Accident and Emergency department
  - 'brittle' asthma
- psychosocial features
- non-compliance with treatment and/or appointments

- poor contact with GP
- self-discharge from hospital
- psychiatric history, including history of self-harm
- drug or alcohol abuse
- learning difficulties
- social problems (unemployment or low income).

Clinical danger signs

These include the following:
- silent chest
- use of accessory muscles of respiration
- brief fragmented speech
- inability to lie in a supine position
- profound sweating
- agitation
- severe symptoms that fail to improve with treatment
- hypotension
- arrhythmias.

Tiring respiratory effort, cyanosis and decreased conscious level are warning signs that respiratory arrest is imminent.

Raised CO_2 levels indicate that the patient requires urgent intubation and ventilation.

Failure of response to treatment together with severe features indicates that consideration should be given to intubation before more life-threatening features develop.

Clinical assessment

Clinical assessment is aimed at identifying the features of severe and life-threatening asthma, as well as looking for alternative diagnoses.

Differential diagnoses
- Pneumothorax:
  — look for any tracheal deviation/lateralising signs.
- Pneumonia/chest infection:
  — local rather than general wheeze or infective sputum.

- Upper airway obstruction:
  — inspiratory stridor rather than expiratory wheeze.

Adjuncts to clinical assessment
Peak expiratory flow (PEF) or FEV$_1$

PEF can be used to assess the severity of the episode and also to monitor the response to treatment. It is most helpful if used as a percentage
of the patient's best normal values, but can also be used as a percentage of the predicted value if the patient's best values are not known (*see*
Table 28.1).

TABLE 28.1 Predicted peak expiratory flow (ml/l)

AGE (YEARS)	FEMALE			MALE		
	HEIGHT (CM) APPROX					
	140	165	190	152	177	207
20	390	460	529	554	649	740
30	380	448	516	532	622	710
40	370	436	502	509	596	680
50	360	424	488	486	569	649

Pulse oximetry

Patients with acute severe asthma may be (but are not always) hypoxae-
mic. Good oxygen saturation levels do not mean that they do not have
severe asthma. The aim of oxygen therapy is to maintain saturations of
94–98%.

Arterial blood gas (ABG) analysis

Patients who show any features of life-threatening asthma, or whose oxygen
saturations are less than 92% on air or oxygen, require an ABG measurement, as do any patients with severe asthma that is not responding to
initial treatment. Saturations of less than 92% are associated with a risk
of developing hypercapnia. A raised arterial carbon dioxide level is a sign
that the patient is tiring and is in imminent danger of respiratory/cardiac
arrest. Carbon dioxide levels will often be low (due to tachypnoea) or within
normal ranges even in patients with life-threatening asthma.

Indications for chest X-ray

- Suspected pneumothorax or pneumomediastinum
- Suspected consolidation
- Life-threatening asthma
- Failure to respond to treatment satisfactorily
- Requirement for ventilation

TABLE 28.2 Features and management of acute severe asthma

FEATURES	TREATMENT
Acute severe asthma	
PEF 35–50% of best or predicted values Respiratory rate 0.25 breaths/min Heart rate 110 beats/min Inability to complete sentences in one breath	Inform senior colleague Salbutamol nebulised at 5 mg 1- to 2-hourly Ipratropium nebulised at 0.5 mg 4- to 6-hourly Prednisolone 40 mg daily or hydrocortisone 100 mg four times a day Aim for oxygen saturation of 94–98% ABG with or without chest X-ray
Life-threatening asthma	
Altered conscious level PEF < 33% of best or predicted values Exhaustion $SpO_2 < 92\%$ $PaO_2 < 8\,kPa$ Arrhythmia Hypotension Normal CO_2 Cyanosis Silent chest Poor respiratory effort *or* acute severe asthma not responding to treatment	**Consider the need for intubation or ventilation** **Involve senior colleague** Salbutamol nebuliser every 15–30 minutes or continuously Continue ipratropium/steroid treatment In addition to the above, consider: Magnesium 1.2–2 g infusion Aminophylline loading dose plus infusion
Near fatal asthma	
Raised $PaCO_2$ Requiring mechanical ventilation with raised inflation pressures	Intubate and ventilate urgently (if patient is not already intubated) In addition to the above, consider: Adrenaline (IV, infusion, SC or ETT), volatile anaesthetic, ketamine infusion

Initial treatment

Oxygen

- Aim for oxygen saturations of 94–98% (remember that these are asthmatic patients, not COPD patients).
- All nebulisers should be oxygen driven, not air driven.

β_2-Agonist bronchodilators

- Salbutamol 5 mg nebulisers can be given every 15–30 minutes.
- The patient can be continuously nebulised at 5–10 mg/hour if equipment is available.
- Intravenous salbutamol can be given in ventilated patients or those in extremis, but has not been shown to be more effective than nebulisers.
- The dose is initially 5 mcg/minute peripherally (range 3–20 mcg/minute).

Ipratropium bromide

- This is nebulised at 0.5 mg every 4–6 hours.
- It is very effective in combination with salbutamol nebulisers in patients with severe asthma.

Steroids

- The oral route is as effective as the parenteral one.
- Give either prednisolone 40 mg daily or hydrocortisone 100 mg 6-hourly.

Intravenous fluids

- These patients often require fluid replacement secondary to poor intake and excessive diaphoresis.

Treatment initiated after consultation with senior staff

This is indicated if there is no response to the above treatments.

Magnesium sulphate

- Give IV magnesium sulphate peripherally as a 1.2–2.0 g infusion over 20 minutes.

Aminophylline infusion

- This is generally not more effective than standard treatment.
- Give an IV 5 mg/kg loading dose over 20 minutes (omit this if the patient is on oral theophylline).
- The loading dose is followed by infusion at a rate of 0.5–0.7 mg/kg/hour.

Treatment used in extremis or if there is difficulty with mechanical ventilation

Adrenaline

- This can be given as a 1 ml bolus (1: 10 000) or as an infusion. It should only be used if the patient is in extremis after failure of the treatment described above. There is a high risk of arrhythmias. Adrenaline can also be given subcutaneously or via an endotracheal tube.

Anaesthetic inhalational agents

- If the appropriate equipment is available, these can be used if all other treatments fail.

Ketamine

- This is a sedative/anaesthetic agent that is given as a bolus or infusion.

Treatments that are not clinically recommended

Antibiotics

- Usually there is a viral trigger, so antibiotics are not needed.

Heliox

- There is no evidence of the efficacy of this mixture of helium and oxygen in asthmatic patients.

Leukotriene receptor antagonists

- There is insufficient evidence of the efficacy of these drugs in asthmatic patients.

Ventilation

Non-invasive ventilation

- There is limited evidence available, but non-invasive ventilation may be beneficial in some patients.
- It is unlikely to benefit patients who are tired or who have raised carbon dioxide levels.
- More randomised controlled trials are needed to identify patients who would benefit from this treatment.

Invasive ventilation

- Patients with severe bronchospasm are often very difficult to ventilate.
- Only small tidal volumes may be possible due to high airway pressures.

'Gas trapping'

- Due to bronchospasm, it is difficult for gas to leave the alveoli. This leads to progressively higher airway pressures with decreasing tidal volumes, and an increased risk of pneumothorax.
- Gas trapping can be countered by allowing adequate expiratory time between breaths.
- The positive end-expiratory pressure (PEEP) usually needs to be low or zero in these patients.
- 'Permissive hypercapnia' is often required, as in ARDS patients.

Further reading

- British Thoracic Society. *Guideline on the Management of Acute Asthma.* London: British Thoracic Society; 2009. www.brit-thoracic.org.uk

29

Burns: ongoing management

Thomas Owen

Inhalation injury

- Diagnosis is most commonly made by bronchoscopy, which gives twice the detection rate that is achieved using clinical findings alone.
- The mainstay of care is to ensure secretion clearance by means of the following:
  — coughing
  — chest physiotherapy
  — airway suctioning
  — therapeutic bronchoscopy.
- The following nebulisers are also used:
  — β2-agonists
  — N-acetylcysteine (20%, 3 ml 4-hourly)
  — heparin (500 U with 3 ml of normal saline).
- ARDS often develops. Use normal ARDS ventilation strategies.
- Ventilator-associated pneumonia (VAP) is also common, and can be difficult to diagnose (*see* Infection section below).
  — Suspect VAP if there is worsening oxygenation.

— Regular broncho-alveolar lavage (BAL) may help to diagnose the condition.
- Patients also often present with carbon monoxide (CO) poisoning.
  — Neurological symptoms occur at CO levels greater than 30%, although there is no clear dose–response relationship.
  — CO poisoning is often difficult to assess, as the patient will have been receiving oxygen (which decreases the half-life of CO) for some time prior to the levels being checked.
  — The role of hyperbaric therapy is not clear, but it may reduce cognitive sequelae in patients with symptomatic poisoning.

Fluid management

- Oedema is worst during the first 24–48 hours.
- Too much fluid exacerbates oedema, whereas too little fluid increases the risk of organ dysfunction. It is difficult to gauge what is just enough!
- The Parkland formula tends to underestimate fluid requirements, but it is easy to over-resuscitate during the first hours ('fluid creep').
- Although the benefits are not proven, the use of cardiac output monitoring and pre-load markers (SVV, etc.) would seem to be logical.
- The choice of fluid is controversial, as no specific advantage has been found for crystalloid or colloid.
- There should be a high level of suspicion for compartment syndromes due to oedema (including abdominal compartment syndrome).

Nutrition/immunotherapy

- The hypermetabolic state can increase the basal metabolic rate (BMR) by 200%.
- Early enteral nutrition is best.
- These patients have increased protein requirements, but high-calorie feeding is not beneficial.
- The addition of glutamine and high-dose vitamin C may be beneficial.
- There is a high risk of stress ulceration, so prophylaxis with a PPI is needed.

Infection

- This is difficult to diagnose.
  - Pyrexia, tachycardia and tachypnoea can persist for months.
  - Suspect infection if new organ dysfunction, decreasing platelet counts and/or increasing fluid requirements are observed.
- Assume that the infection is related to the central line until proven otherwise.

Rhabdomyolysis

This condition is most commonly seen with the following:
- extensive burns
- electrical burns
- trauma
- drug overdose
- prolonged immobilisation.

Diagnosis

- High index of suspicion
- Creatine kinase (CK) level 5–10 times the normal value
- Myoglobin in urine (dipstick positive for blood in the absence of red blood cells) – not always positive
- Hyperkalaemia
- Acute renal failure

Treatment

- Assess and treat for compartment syndromes.
- Maintain a high urine output to 'flush out' myoglobin.
  - Aim for a rate of 200–300 ml/hour.
  - Consider mannitol when the patient is adequately hydrated.
- Alkalinise the urine to prevent precipitation of myoglobin. Aim for a urinary pH of > 6, using either of the following:
  - sodium bicarbonate
  - acetazolamide.

30

Organ donation in critical care

Huw Twamley

Cadaveric (as opposed to living) organ donation can be classified as follows:
- heart-beating donation
- non-heart-beating donation
- tissue donation.

Heart-beating or brainstem-dead donation
Brainstem death occurs when the brainstem herniates through the foramen magnum, disrupting the blood supply (a process which is also known as 'coning'). This results in irreversible loss of brainstem function.

Functions of the brainstem
These include the following:
- consciousness/awareness
- respiratory drive
- endocrine regulation
- cranial nerve function
- *cardiac central regulation* (the heart continues to beat due to intrinsic rhythm rather than central control).

Loss of brainstem function inevitably leads to cardiac arrest in all patients within hours or days. This is **not** the same as persistent vegetative state, which is loss of cerebral function and has a variable prognosis.

Brainstem death is legally the same as cardiorespiratory death, as it is 'the irreversible loss of consciousness in addition to the irreversible loss of the capacity to breathe.'

Diagnosis and testing for cessation of brainstem function
This is performed by two doctors, who should fulfil the following criteria.
- They should both have been registered for at least 5 years.
- One of them should be a consultant.
- They should be competent in brainstem testing.
- They should be independent of the donation team.

Inclusion criteria
- Known aetiology of unconsciousness.
- Fully ventilated patient.
- Fixed unresponsive pupils.

Exclusion criteria
- Depressant drugs: the length of time between discontinuation of depressant drugs and undertaking brainstem testing depends on several factors, including the nature of the drug, total dose, duration of treatment, and the renal and hepatic function.
- Neuromuscular blocking drugs.
- Hypothermia (< 34 °C).
- Metabolic or endocrine disturbances.

Tests for absence of brainstem function
1 Do the pupils react to light?
2 Are there corneal reflexes (elicited by lightly touching the cornea with a wisp of cotton wool)?
3 Is there eye movement on calorific testing (i.e. is there any nystagmus on instillation of ice cold saline into the external auditory meatus)?
4 Is there a motor response to painful stimulation in the facial area, limbs or trunk (supraorbital pressure, nail bed pressure, sternal pressure)?

5 Is there a gag reflex (i.e. palate movement in response to tongue depressor)?

6 Is there a cough reflex (stimulated by suctioning via a tracheal tube)?

Apnoea test (respiratory response to hypercarbia)

* Increase the FiO_2 to 1.0 to pre-oxygenate.
* Reduce minute ventilation until the $PaCO_2$ is > 6.0 kPa *and* the pH is < 7.4 (arterial blood gases). (If the patient is a CO_2 retainer, allow a higher $PaCO_2$ until the pH is < 7.4.)
* Disconnect the patient from the ventilator while instilling 100% oxygen via a suction catheter.
* Look for any respiratory movements for 5 minutes. Oxygen saturation must be above 95%.
* After 5 minutes, check that the $PaCO_2$ has risen by at least 0.5 kPa (check arterial blood gases).

Summary

* Two complete sets of tests must be performed (the legal time of death is when the first set of tests indicates death due to the absence of brain-stem reflexes).
* There is no rule stating the time interval that is required between tests. The second set of tests is often performed immediately after the first.
* Consent must be obtained from the patient's next of kin.
* The **legally dead patient** is then taken to theatre for organ retrieval.
* It is possible to donate heart, lungs, liver, pancreas, kidneys and intestine if suitable.

Non-heart-beating donation

* Potential donors are those patients in whom critical care treatment is withdrawn because its continuation is considered to be futile.
* If the family consents, the retrieval team are ready in theatre at the point of withdrawal (in critical care).
* If the patient dies within 2 hours of withdrawal, they are taken quickly to theatre.
* Cold perfusion of the kidneys and liver is started within 10 minutes of cardiorespiratory death.

- It is possible to donate kidneys, liver, and occasionally pancreas and lungs.

Tissue donation

- This occurs post-mortem.
- It is possible to donate corneas, heart valves, bone, skin, and ligaments/ tendons.

Further reading

- Academy of Medical Royal Colleges. *A Code of Practice for the Diagnosis and Confirmation of Death.* London: Academy of Medical Royal Colleges; 2008.

Index